Dr John Gedney qualified from the University of Nottingham in 1979 and from 1984 worked as a GP in Northumberland with a special interest in mental health, rheumatic diseases and diabetes. Now retired from clinical work he has an ongoing interest in the challenges posed by people being overweight and the pandemic of type 2 diabetes, particularly in the context of the food environment and the evolving science of metabolic syndrome.

Pamela Myles-Hooton worked as an accredited cognitive behavioural therapist for over twenty years and is an honorary fellow of the British Association for Behavioural and Cognitive Psychotherapies (BABCP). She wrote *How to Beat Agoraphobia* and co-wrote *The CBT Handbook*. She spent over eleven years training others in delivering evidence-based psychological interventions at the University of Reading, and later worked with NHS Education for Scotland to develop a training programme for mental health staff who help people experiencing anxiety and depression.

T0384357

Living Well self-help guides use clinically proven techniques
to treat long-standing and disabling conditions,
both psychological and physical.

Series Editors: Professor Kate Harvey and
Emeritus Professor Peter Cooper

Books in the *Living Well* series

Living Well Through the Menopause

Living Well with Tinnitus

LIVING WELL WITH TYPE 2 DIABETES

John Gedney, Pamela Myles-Hooton

ROBINSON

ROBINSON

First published in Great Britain in 2024 by Robinson

1 3 5 7 9 10 8 6 4 2

Important Note
This book is not intended as a substitute for medical advice or treatment.
Any person with a condition requiring medical attention should consult a
qualified medical practitioner or suitable therapist.

A CIP catalogue record for this book
is available from the British Library.

ISBN: 978-1-47214-601-4

Typeset in Berkeley by Initial Typesetting Services, Edinburgh
Printed and bound in Great Britain by Clays Ltd, Elcograf S.p.A.

Papers used by Robinson are from well-managed forests
and other responsible sources.

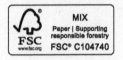

MIX
Paper | Supporting
responsible forestry
FSC® C104740

Robinson
An imprint of
Little, Brown Book Group
Carmelite House
50 Victoria Embankment
London EC4Y 0DZ

An Hachette UK Company
www.hachette.co.uk

www.littlebrown.co.uk

Contents

Section IV
Type 2 diabetes and psychological wellbeing

Introduction: about type 2 diabetes

'I was in my late thirties when I went to see my doctor. I was absolutely exhausted, utterly lacking energy. I didn't feel ill but neither did I feel well. I'm not sure what I was expecting – everyone says they are tired these days, don't they? I was convinced I was lacking something. We talked about my steady weight gain since having our daughter Chloe, then aged six. The doctor examined me and then said it was a good idea to do some simple blood tests. He could see that I'd had pregnancy diabetes when I was carrying Chloe, and I was embarrassed to say I'd not followed up the reminders about getting it regularly checked. We agreed it was a good idea to test for that too.'

Suzanne, 47

Suzanne's tests showed that she was not lacking anything but that she was 'at risk' of type 2 diabetes (T2D). A few months later, after losing weight, her test results were back to normal. She later developed type 2 diabetes during a stressful time in her life and we'll follow some of her journey throughout the book. Her story demonstrates so many of the features of T2D and how they get caught up with the twists and turns of life.

Suzanne was at risk of T2D partly because her mother had the disease and pregnancy had then simply highlighted that additional risk. After the pregnancy came lasting weight gain, eventually tipping her into T2D. On the earlier occasion, when deemed at risk of T2D, then later when she developed the disease, she managed to lose weight *and* reverse the changes of T2D. By keeping her weight stable, she was then able to continue in remission – free of T2D.

Research suggests that up to 50 per cent of people diagnosed with T2D can put their condition into remission by changing the way they live – especially the way they eat. Even without getting T2D into full-on 'reverse gear', similar lifestyle changes can still improve the condition, making better health – and perhaps less medication – within the reach of many more people. It requires a determined mindset and hard work to get back your health, but it can be done, and many have achieved it.

There are three principles that thread their way through this book:

- The first is that you need relevant and up-to-date knowledge to tackle T2D.

- The second is that you will need to find and hold on to your innermost motivation to achieve the changes to help you manage your T2D.

- And the third is – with help – to find those ways of living, especially around eating, that work for *you*.

This book is about giving you that knowledge and encouraging that determined mindset but also being realistic about the hard work which will be needed long-term to stay well.

A diagnosis of T2D may have come as a surprise or even a shock to you, and is likely to be impacting your daily life. You may sense an impending change in your life or be worried that something bad may happen. Some of your fears may be realistic, but of course human nature is often to imagine the worst, which can make starting to fight back that bit harder – at least to begin with. This book will help you to understand T2D, avoid it if you are at risk and, if you have it, to try to understand *why* it may have happened to you. We will set out how best to live well with T2D and possibly even 'reverse' it. The fact that you have opened the book is an important first step in managing your fears, learning about T2D, and about what you can do to reclaim your life.

Who the book is for

This book is mainly intended for people with T2D, and their families or carers. It is highly relevant to people who are most at risk of being diagnosed with T2D, which would be any near relatives, such as a sibling or a child of an affected person. It is also for anyone in follow-up for a previously raised blood glucose reading, including women who have experienced diabetes in pregnancy.

It may also be of interest to healthcare professionals who deal with T2D, including those who work in mental health services.

T2D is becoming much more common and around half of all people in the world are overweight and/or have conditions which relate to T2D, so we could argue that most people could benefit from thinking about the issues we raise in the book!

Why 'self-help' is vital

Self-help is so important in many long-term medical conditions; most gains in health come from what we do for ourselves and with T2D this feels even more vital since we know that:

- As Suzanne demonstrated, T2D can be reversed and put into remission, or substantially improved, by changing the way we eat, and live.

- Equally importantly, T2D can be *prevented* in much the same way.

- Medical management can, to a degree, reduce the risks from having T2D but does not treat the actual *underlying* disease, which goes on regardless.

- Standard nutritional advice has made little, if any, difference to the growing number of people with T2D and we need to understand why.

If you have T2D or are at risk of developing it, healthcare will support and help, but what *you* do to help yourself will ultimately make a far bigger difference – with the biggest gains of all if you can put your T2D into remission.

What's inside?

First of all, before we look at what's inside, we should introduce ourselves and explain a bit about who we are and why we have written this book.

John

I qualified in medicine from the University of Nottingham in 1979, before early professional training in both general practice and hospital medicine. During a thirty-four-year career as a GP I developed a special interest in long-term medical conditions, notably in the fields of rheumatology and diabetes, serving on national working groups in both. I was also involved in developing general practice-based mental health service provision.

Through the middle and later stages of my career, diabetes became my main focus; I wanted to know why type 2 diabetes was becoming so much more common, and why we had assumed it to be a milder form of diabetes, when it was clearly not.

People say it's hard to fix a problem if you don't know what the problem is, and until the last decade, we could say this applied to type 2 diabetes. Though I am now retired from clinical work, my curiosity and commitment to understanding the disease continue undiminished.

Pam

Originally from Scotland, I am author/co-author of several educational texts, academic publications and self-help books, including *The CBT Handbook* and *How to Beat Agoraphobia*. I contributed to Health Education England's curriculum for low-intensity practitioners working with people with long-term physical health conditions. I sit on the NHS Talking Therapies for Anxiety and Depression Expert Advisory Group.

For over twenty years I worked as a cognitive behavioural therapist, mainly in the NHS. Overlapping with this work, I led the development and delivery of cognitive behavioural therapy training programmes at the University of Reading for eleven years. More recently I worked with NHS Education for Scotland to develop a training programme for mental health staff who help people experiencing anxiety and depression. In 2020, I became one of three directors of Bespoke Mental Health, which provides online training in evidence-based psychological treatments for mental health practitioners and operates as not-for-profit for the NHS and charities.

We will begin with a brief outline of T2D, and the experience of being diagnosed with the condition.

Section I (Chapters 1–4) is all about preparing you for the challenge of T2D, first by helping you to understand just what the disease is all about – and showing how far our thinking has moved on in the last decade. We'll see why it's important to become – and stay – physically active, and why good sleep matters in preventing and managing T2D. We will look at how different people approach T2D after being diagnosed, and the value of motivation and an effective mindset in tackling it.

Section II (Chapters 5 and 6) is mainly about food and the way we eat. We'll be covering the current 'hot topic' of reversing T2D and the equally important subject of how best to eat long-term for T2D. Robust scientific evidence is gathering around reversal, but that's quite new, and we don't have the experience yet of how best to follow up on reversal and hold the disease in long-term remission. We do, however, have good evidence for a small number of dietary approaches which improve T2D and these will be the focus of what we call 'eating for the long haul' – that is, for life.

In Section III (Chapters 7, 8 and 9), we'll look at the risks of T2D and how to reduce them by being more in control, using knowledge, self-monitoring and self-management to improve T2D. Self-monitoring of blood glucose helps a proportion of people, but we think it could help more, with better under-standing and more support from healthcare teams.

Almost everyone should monitor their own blood pressure, and we will make a case too for purposeful monitoring of any problem area – whether it be around eating, or tracking sleep, mood or exercise. Self-monitoring helps us to stay engaged and more in control of our body – and almost certainly helps us to improve our health.

In Chapter 9, we'll take a look at T2D and pregnancy. Reproduction is nature's way of passing on the best of us, but with a disease like T2D, some not-so-good things can be passed on too. Both T2D and (the related) pregnancy or gestational diabetes are now the commonest forms of diabetes in pregnancy, reflecting the surge in T2D in younger people all around the world.

It's beginning to look like genetics is more complex than any of us could have realised. Being at risk of T2D carries not only increased risks to mother and infant during the pregnancy, but also additional and enduring risks to children even well into adult life. Transmission of disease across generations may underpin some of the rapid growth in T2D generally and we'll try to explain why this is an issue for all adults, not just for pregnant women.

When we look at how the body works, and how T2D develops, we can see that all the systems of the body are involved – things connect. If the brain is involved then the mind is too, and T2D demonstrates just how joined up mind and body really are.

In Section IV (Chapters 10 and 11), we will explore how psychological issues, mental health problems and T2D can interact – and what you can do to help yourself.

We will close, then, with a summary of key points from the book and an update on the onward journeys of our T2D case examples, introduced below and in Chapter 1.

How to use the book

Read the book however you wish, as the chapter titles and short summary notes at the end of each chapter can help you navigate around. However, we would recommend reading Section I first, where we start by getting a feel for T2D and how things work; current science might just challenge some of your thinking about this disease.

Case examples

Our case examples, introduced fully in Chapter 1, will illustrate some of the common experiences and feelings people have at the outset with T2D. Though experiences are real, names and identifying features have, of course, been changed or removed.

We will revisit these people throughout the book. You have briefly met Suzanne, and will soon get to know others such as Mustafa, who developed T2D when working night shifts; Margaret, whose journey started with a visit to her optician; Ted, who had high blood pressure; and Nandita, whose T2D was diagnosed after developing odd sensations in her hands. What they all have in common is T2D and some of their experiences may be relevant to you.

Signposting

The world of T2D is a big one and it overlaps particularly with body weight and nutrition. We have already said that most of the good that gets done is by people themselves, not by professionals and healthcare teams. We'll put more emphasis, therefore, on exploring behaviours and choices.

And if you want to know more, we will signpost to other materials in the appendices at the end of the book. There are some great sources and inspirational stories out there!

References, terminology, other resources such as diaries, and further reading suggestions can be found at the end of the book.

About T2D

We associate diabetes with the pancreas – where insulin is made – and with too much glucose in the blood, which is the hallmark of diabetes generally. With T2D however, the disease is not caused simply by a lack of insulin (as happens in type 1 diabetes). Indeed, for the most part the body is producing *more* insulin than usual. 'Behind the scenes' of T2D lies a fault in the way the body is storing and using its two main fuels – glucose and fat. This problem involves not just the pancreas but the two main organs of energy control within the body, the brain and liver, and the way insulin itself is working. A better understanding of what has been going wrong with insulin takes us to the very heart of T2D.

Doctors have typically concentrated on lowering blood glucose, and we have long had the tools (medications) to do this. We also know that lowering glucose lowers the risks from T2D – at least up to a point. It is no surprise then that the medical focus has been on glucose itself. But this approach does not address the *reason* for blood glucose going up in the first place, nor correct other harmful and important changes in the body's chemistry which also define T2D, and probably even more of its risks.

Addressing these things is where you come in!

Science can now explain much more about how T2D comes about, and although not everything is within our control, some important things are, especially what and how we choose to eat. If we can *really* change the way we fuel our body, it is possible to improve or restore normal insulin function. And if we can do that we will see weight loss, and more importantly normal blood glucose, and the restoration of health. *This* is the main treatment of T2D itself.

For sure, being healthy is about more than just food, but we can say that living well *with* T2D is *mainly* about eating well *for* T2D.

There are now around half a billion people with T2D in the world. It affects one in fifteen people and has undergone a fivefold increase over forty years. It is associated with being overweight, but T2D is increasing proportionately faster than are the rates of being overweight or obese – alarming though they are. In Europe and North America, between 5 and 10 per cent of people are affected, and in lower- and middle-income countries the figures are even higher. Between a quarter and a third of all people affected by T2D live in China, where little more than a generation ago the disease was almost unknown.

Wherever you live, you probably know someone with T2D.

We want to help reduce the number of people with T2D, and the number of people who suffer a serious problem as a result of having T2D – starting with *you*.

Introducing type 2 diabetes

Colin, 62, carpenter

Colin has recently been in hospital after a heart attack. He had been surprised at how little it had affected him, and had started to think himself lucky until the hospital doctor told him that he had T2D – and his blood pressure was higher than it should be. He had been feeling low, worrying about possible redundancies at work, and had been sleeping badly for months. He was constantly tired. He and his wife talked a lot about 'stress'.

Colin was seeing his local healthcare team for follow-up checks and next-step planning. He'd felt thoroughly miserable since leaving hospital – all he could think about were money worries and now, with uncertain future health, he wondered 'what the point of it all was'. He would later recall that this was an all-time low. His wife had worked very hard to get him to his appointment. She thought his stress and low mood had 'brought everything on'. She was anxious about the future too.

In the last few decades, fewer people smoking and better, quicker treatment of heart attacks has meant fewer people dying from heart disease. But like the fairground whack-a-mole game, just as you think you are getting one problem down, another pops up in its place!

A significant proportion of people admitted to hospital with a heart attack are found to have one or more features of metabolic syndrome, which include hypertension (high blood pressure) and T2D. As we move through the first section of the book, we'll see how T2D is not just about too much glucose in the blood but involves a range of changes in metabolism, which impact health much more.

Colin has T2D and he has metabolic syndrome – a term used by doctors and scientists to describe how T2D sits within a wider cluster of related health conditions.

What is diabetes?

Diabetes is short for diabetes mellitus (DM) – a mixture of Greek and Latin words. Diabetes means 'syphon' – the movement of fluid or water – because a classic diabetes symptom is peeing a lot. Mellitus means 'honeyed' or 'sweet' – referring to the characteristic sweetness of the urine in diabetes. In ancient times, physicians really would diagnose diabetes by tasting their patients' urine (no dipsticks!). To have too much glucose in the urine, a person has too much glucose in the bloodstream, which then spills over into the urine when blood is filtered by the kidneys. So behind some of the typical symptoms of diabetes is an abnormally high level of glucose in the bloodstream – **hyperglycaemia** is the medical term.

What actually is T2D?

The two most common reasons for persisting hyperglycaemia are type 1 diabetes (T1D) and T2D. In spite of the hyperglycaemia which gives each its name they have less in common than you might imagine!

In the first half of the last century, there was still no official separation of the types of diabetes – though doctors noticed that their older patients tended to carry more weight, and when insulin was introduced in the 1920s, they showed little or no response to the new treatment which was keeping their younger, slimmer patients alive. Later, when it became possible to measure insulin levels in the blood, it was clear that people with T2D did not always lack insulin – indeed many had *elevated* levels.

T1D and T2D are different and separate conditions

The legacy of calling all instances of raised blood glucose diabetes is that we tend to see them as more alike than they really are. T1D and T2D don't have the same cause, or behave in the same way, and outcomes – though similar – are not the same. They really are different diseases, which happen to overlap because of hyperglycaemia.

A common question is, 'I have type 2 diabetes, but am now on insulin – does this mean I now have type 1 diabetes?' No! T2D is a different disease, whether treated with insulin or not. Using insulin to lower blood glucose says nothing about the underlying nature of the condition. *Everyone* with T1D uses insulin because they need it to stay alive; insulin is lost quite quickly and permanently – injections replace the missing natural insulin. Until the late stages of the disease, *lack* of insulin is not the problem in T2D, which develops against a backdrop of *higher than usual* insulin levels. But although insulin is present, the way that it regulates blood glucose has become defective, a state generally called **insulin resistance**. In Chapter 2 we will see how this problem plays a key role in bringing about T2D. With T1D, insulin is absent and with T2D, insulin is often present but not working as it should.

Although increasing numbers of young people are being diagnosed with T2D, it is still a disease which is more likely to appear in mid-life and beyond. By contrast, the average age of onset of T1D is around thirteen years. T2D also evolves more slowly, typically taking years or even decades to fully surface. A person with T2D is usually less visibly ill, that is unless you are a 'Colin' and suffer a heart attack before you even realised you had T2D. T1D presents with weight loss – often profound – whereas with T2D there is nearly always weight *gain*.

The conundrum of T2D is that it has always looked mild – indeed people called it 'mild diabetes' – but now we can see that it is far from mild. T2D affects older people because the impact of insulin resistance is slow. It is also what makes a person susceptible to high blood pressure, heart attacks, stroke and poor (limb) circulation. They are not so much complications of T2D but part of its very nature.

Around 95 per cent of people with ongoing diabetes have T2D.

Figure 1.1: T1D and T2D overlap – but less than you might think

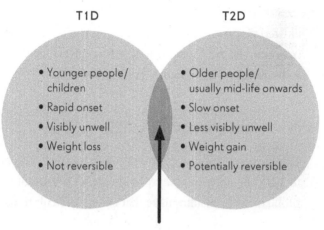

Both show raised blood glucose and similar
(but not the same) complications

T1D and T2D look different because they *are* different.

How does T2D show itself?

T2D is a complex condition that evolves slowly, usually over years. To begin with many people have no symptoms, or changes are so gradual that they are not experienced as abnormal. Eventually most people do experience noticeable symptoms – broadly of two kinds:

Those of hyperglycaemia

- Peeing a lot, thirst, and genital soreness and itching from recurring fungal infections – both sexes; this is glucose 'overspill' into the urine.

- Blurred vision – caused by a changing glucose concentration in the eye fluids, which in turn affects focusing. It disappears when glucose levels settle.

And those of the wider effects of T2D

- Tiredness – a real lack of energy affects nearly everyone in T2D; the body has plenty of energy on board but problems with insulin make that energy difficult to use.

- Hunger is common in T2D, and is caused by disturbances in the hormones – including insulin – which regulate appetite.

- Weight gain is almost ever-present in T2D, and the gain is usually long-term, over years.

Surprisingly perhaps, slimmer people can also develop T2D – though their weight gain is typically less.

Hyperglycaemia is usually less pronounced in T2D than in T1D, so those connected 'classical' diabetes symptoms may be mild, barely noticeable or even absent.

T2D can come to attention at any point, and detected early it's often when a person is having a check-up for another problem such as high blood pressure. Following up previous borderline glucose values, routine medical checks, such as those related to employment or insurance issues, can also reveal early T2D.

Suggestive symptoms or the investigation of a problem, like Colin's heart attack, may also reveal underlying T2D.

Here's how T2D came into the lives of some of the people we know:

Ted, 78, retired

Ted was seeing the nurse for a review of his blood pressure and mentioned that he had been peeing a bit more, getting up two or three times at night rather than his usual once. He had put it down to age or his prostate. He felt fine otherwise. It had not crossed his mind that he could have diabetes. Diagnosis of T2D over the age of seventy-five does not pose the same problems and risks as it would if it appeared earlier in life. If managed sensibly, it may impact little on quality or length of life.

T2D coming on later in life can feel 'mild'.

Cassie, 56, estate agent

Cassie had been progressively unwell for several months when she was diagnosed with T2D. Something of a lifelong exerciser, with a lean athletic build, she had been running and swimming regularly until a dramatic loss of energy brought her to a standstill. She was passing urine much more than usual and suffered repeated infections. She was no one's idea of a candidate for T2D and the diagnosis was a big shock to those that knew her and to Cassie herself.

T2D can occur in slim, previously fit people.

Suzanne, 47, secretary

Suzanne visited her doctor at the age of thirty-eight reporting tiredness and mild diarrhoea. She had slowly gained weight following the birth of her daughter six years before. Her mum had T2D. Her blood tests showed mildly abnormal liver function and that she herself was at risk of T2D.

After a few months of substantial weight loss, she no longer felt tired, and her blood tests returned to normal. Planned checkups for one reason or another did not happen and after two years, the family moved away because of her husband's job.

The house move did not go especially well and Suzanne felt isolated, using alcohol to help mask her anxiety and to sleep. Later, her symptoms and weight gain returned, and she was diagnosed with T2D five years after the first borderline test results. She regretted not seeking further help in the interim but just lacked the motivation, saying she had 'put her head in the sand'.

We will see later (Chapter 9) how family issues motivated Suzanne to enable her to regain control of her health.

T2D can develop when life gets in the way of us looking after ourselves.

Mustafa, 54, factory worker

Mustafa, originally from Iraq, works in a car factory in the UK. He developed raised blood pressure in his forties and was in annual medical review. Nearing fifty, he began to work a rotating shift pattern at work. Soon after, he began to feel excessively tired, experiencing both weight gain and difficulty controlling his blood pressure. His regular checks revealed that he had developed T2D.

Within five years of being diagnosed he had needed insulin treatment to achieve reasonable blood glucose control, along with multiple medications for his blood pressure.

We will come back to Mustafa in Chapter 4 when we look at the impact of disturbed sleep on how the body works, and how this might worsen a person's T2D journey. We will also use his experience of navigating Ramadan, on insulin, to illustrate the value of self-monitoring of blood glucose (Chapter 8).

Disturbed sleep, whatever its cause, can affect metabolism and potentially worsen or even cause T2D.

Margaret, 62, carer

Apart from developing what she called a 'weak bladder', Margaret felt in good health. But then she developed blurred vision. Her optician was unable to explain her symptoms but her practice nurse found her blood pressure to be elevated. Routine blood tests subsequently revealed T2D.

Margaret had a positive disposition and, whilst disappointed by the news, she was not unduly worried. Her elderly aunt had T2D and had been well enough so far, she reasoned. Margaret felt herself fortunate to be diagnosed before any serious problem had developed. She initially managed dietary reversal of her T2D but struggled to hold on to it, and we'll look at her efforts in Chapters 5 and 6. Margaret's vision and her 'weak bladder' returned to normal when her glucose level improved.

Blurred vision may be explained not by an eye problem, but by a change in a person's blood glucose level.

Benjamin, 55, air traffic controller

Regular work medicals had shown moderate weight gain over a decade before Benjamin was diagnosed with raised blood pressure (hypertension). At the age of fifty-one, he was diagnosed with T2D with no suggestive symptoms other than getting out of bed to pee more often.

Benjamin was born of Jamaican parents, neither of whom had T2D, though both had hypertension; T2D is significantly more common in the Black Caribbean population. He worked in air traffic control, and was anxious about the impact of diabetes on his job – particularly as he would not be allowed to work as a controller if on insulin.

He lost a reasonable amount of weight and had fairly good control of his blood glucose on oral medication. His main ongoing problem was a difficulty adjusting psychologically to his T2D, and ongoing worry about job security.

In some people the impact of T2D can be more psychological.

Nandita, 60, retired teacher

Nandita, whose family were from India, was born in the UK. She was a music teacher but retired early due to neuropathy (pains and loss of feeling in her hands and feet) which interfered with her work. She had always been an anxious person, and this became a problem in itself after she developed T2D with its complications.

Persistent tingling in her hands had taken her to see a doctor, not long after the age of fifty. Slowly rising weight, urinary symptoms and fatigue suggested that Nandita's T2D had probably been smouldering for a decade, and within five years of diagnosis, she was on insulin. T2D and mental health problems can be so bound up that it's hard to see, looking back, which is the 'chicken' and which is the 'egg' – and this was the case with Nandita.

Enduring anxiety drives the stress hormone system of the body which in turn can contribute to the onset and course of T2D.

Colin

We have already introduced Colin. He suffered the double whammy of experiencing a heart attack and the diagnosis of

T2D at the same time. He had been feeling low for about a year and getting physically unwell had put him in a very bad place. It took a long time for him to adjust and eventually get on top of his health problems. Parts of his journey appear throughout the book.

T2D can smoulder on in the background before coming to light through a major complication.

Here are two people without T2D but with a relevant associated problem:

Chloe, 15, school student

Chloe is Suzanne's daughter. She has not been diagnosed with T2D, but her strong family history (mother and grandmother have T2D) puts her at risk. She herself became overweight in her teens, and was diagnosed with PCOS – polycystic ovary syndrome, which can affect menstrual periods, fertility and body weight, and can cause acne, which affected Chloe quite badly. PCOS is considered to be part of the metabolic syndrome mentioned earlier, and so is linked to T2D. We will explain more about the link and what happened with Chloe in Chapter 9.

We can be at risk of T2D through the complexity of inheritance.

Alan, 42, police officer

Alan, a police inspector, found his weight rising slowly in spite of being active, including jogging up to twenty miles a week. His annual medical check at work showed his blood pressure to be up a little, and his liver function blood test was mildly abnormal. He was found to have a fatty liver (NAFLD – non-alcoholic fatty liver disease), which is strongly connected to T2D.

Alan believed that exercise would keep him fit and healthy, regardless of his dietary and social habits (he liked his beer!), but his rising weight and his liver problem challenged that belief.

We can be at risk of T2D if we follow our beliefs and ignore the facts.

Pause for thought: Your story with T2D

How was your T2D diagnosed? Are there similarities with any of our cases? What have you done so far to help tackle the problem? How successful has that been? Make a note of ongoing problems and, as you work your way through the book, check the advice to see how you might try to tackle them.

Measuring blood glucose, and making sense of HbA1c

Hyperglycaemia – Other than defining diabetes and causing its most recognisable symptoms, a raised blood glucose level has also been our benchmark for judging the severity of T2D and, historically, how to manage it. It's helpful, therefore, to understand how blood glucose is measured and to get a feel for what the numbers mean. You will hopefully get to know your way around glucose testing as we go through the book, and if you are new to T2D, your healthcare team will probably have given you a good start. But we know that even when people have had T2D for a long time, the tests can still confuse, and some basic revision might be useful – especially on HbA1c (more on that later).

Glucose – There are two main ways to assess blood glucose. The first is to simply measure it! If John were to test a sample of Pam's blood at, say 9.45 a.m., he would discover her glucose reading at the time the test was taken. When interpreting the result he would need to know that she ate some porridge and toast at 8 a.m. Blood glucose is an 'in-the-moment' test and to interpret it we need more information, especially the time and content of the last meal. To know what the reading is later in the day, after the next meal or after a walk, etc., would need multiple tests.

Glucose, like most chemicals in the body, is a variable – it changes, and what's more, it changes *continuously*, so any test result is a snapshot from the bigger, *moving* picture of what's actually happening. The same applies to most other tests or measurements. For example, cholesterol, weight, kidney function and blood pressure all change by the moment, and throughout a day. Some things don't change much during a twenty-four-hour period, or the variation matters less. The variation with blood glucose, however, matters a lot; knowing its level on waking (when it's usually lowest) and two hours after eating (when at its highest) tells us how T2D is doing. Multiple tests were once the only way of gauging T2D. Then along came the second way of assessing blood glucose, which is HbA1c.

HbA1c – This test transformed the monitoring of T2D when it came into widespread use in the 1980s. Measuring HbA1c gives a reliable estimation of *average* blood glucose and is the test most often used to assess or even to diagnose T2D. For most people, most of the time, it is the only test they and their healthcare teams use to monitor T2D. Everyone gets used to HbA1c (eventually), but to begin with it can be hard to grasp what it's measuring and what it means. The abbreviation stands for haemoglobin A1c, also sometimes called glycated haemoglobin. Glycation is the word for the chemical attachment of a sugar – in this case glucose, to (usually) a protein – and here it's haemoglobin.

Haemoglobin (Hb) is the important oxygen-carrying protein in all of our red blood cells. We measure Hb to assess the health of the blood generally – a normal Hb level tells you that you are not anaemic.

Measuring *glycated* Hb – HbA1c – in the laboratory gives an indication of how much glucose has been in contact with the red blood cell (and the haemoglobin inside it) during the lifespan of the cell, which is roughly three or four months. The more glucose in the blood, the more it attaches to the Hb, and the higher the HbA1c reading becomes. The HbA1c level therefore reflects indirectly, but accurately, the *average* level of glucose in the bloodstream over a three- to four-month period.

Figure 1.2: The making of haemoglobin A1c (HbA1c)

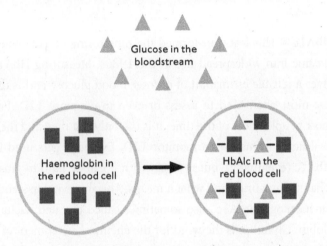

In summary, the two tests of blood glucose in regular use are glucose itself – a snapshot test giving a direct measure of the glucose level at a specific time – and HbA1c, an indirect reflection of average blood glucose over the previous three months – with the variability of individual glucose readings smoothed out.

Here's how these tests can be used when answering the key questions:

Do I have T2D? – Both blood glucose and HbA1c can be used for diagnosing T2D. A blood glucose test would need to be performed in the morning after an overnight fast. Doing both tests is common practice and helps make the diagnosis more secure, though neither is infallible.

How's my blood glucose doing? – Either just in general, or for example since making a change such as cutting back on food after Christmas. These 'How are things going generally?' questions need a HbA1c test. A single – or even a few – blood glucose readings would not be enough. HbA1c checked every 4–6 months, or 3–4 months after making a lifestyle/diet change is a standard and reliable way of tracking blood glucose indirectly in T2D.

What happens to my blood glucose when I eat a loaded bagel? – This is a different, more 'here-and-now' sort of question. To answer this, you would want to measure your blood glucose before and after eating the bagel. HbA1c would not help you here – the impact of the bagel, even several bagels, on your HbA1c would be too small and feedback too slow to be useful.

People who self-monitor (see Chapter 8) use HbA1c to track their T2D path overall, and use blood glucose readings to assess the day-to-day impact of treatments, particularly insulin, and of illness. Assessing the impact of lifestyle changes – taking up a new exercise, changing a shift-work pattern or the impact of bagels! – can be done over a few days tracking blood glucose, and over weeks or months with HbA1c.

Don't worry if HbA1c confuses you. Many people struggle with it, but it is *the* main test in assessing T2D and it's worth spending time on. A link to an audio-visual explanation of HbA1c is in Appendix 2: Terminology (for Chapter 1). There's more on the subject in Chapter 8 too.

The units for expressing blood glucose and HbA1c

Apologies, this is dull but might be useful!

Blood glucose is expressed in mmol/L (millimoles per litre) – this is the modern standard, used for example in Canada, the UK, China, Australasia and half of Europe.

Or mg/dL (milligrams per decilitre), used in the US, South America, India/southern Asia and the other half of Europe!

HbA1c can be expressed in mmol/mol (millimoles per mole). Again, the modern standard and generally used where glucose is expressed in mmol/L units.

Or as a percentage (the proportion of Hb that has glucose attached). Mainly used in the US.

Confusingly, some countries use old units for glucose and newer units for HbA1c, or even both at the same time!

The numbers themselves (old and new units) relating to a diagnosis of T2D

If you have been diagnosed with T2D, you will have had a fasting glucose reading of at least 7mmol/L (126mg/dL). Normal levels are usually around 4–6mmol/L (72–108mg/dL). If you have been diagnosed with T2D following a HbA1c test, the result will have been 48mmol/mol (6.5%) or higher, ideally done more than once.

You only need to become familiar with the units in your own country – and remember that glucose and HbA1c, while connected, are not the same thing; their units are different and the range of numbers is different. Be mindful of the unit differences if reading guidance or articles from other countries online.

> **Pause for thought**
>
> Can you remember your HbA1c reading at diagnosis? How has it changed since?

Here are the first HbA1c readings for some of our case examples:

	HbA1c – mmol/mol (%)
Colin	64 (8.0%)
Margaret	60 (7.6%)
Suzanne	52 (6.9%)
Cassie	104 (11.7%)
Ted	56 (7.3%)
Mustafa	50 (6.7%)
Benjamin	55 (7.2%)
Nandita	60 (7.6%)

They all had mild symptoms except Cassie, who was really very unwell; a HbA1c of 104 (11.7%) meant that her average blood glucose would have been around three times the normal!

Colin suffered a heart attack before he knew he had T2D, so you might be surprised that his HbA1c was only 64 (8%). It's still worth bearing in mind that, although this sounds like a modest elevation of HbA1c, it correlates with an average blood glucose which is twice normal.

In Chapter 8 we'll look more at how the values of blood glucose and HbA1c connect with each other.

Figure 1.3: What on earth has happened with T2D?

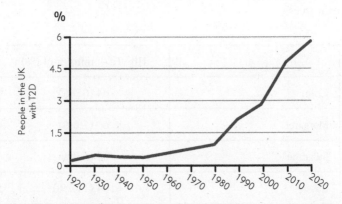

Though based on UK data, the graph in Figure 1.3 would look similar in most countries. The slope might be either a little flatter or steeper, or be a year or two in front or behind, but it would still be there.

The rise in T2D since the 1980s is unprecedented for a non-infectious disease. T1D has increased a little during this period, but the vast majority of the rise in numbers has been from T2D. We have become so used to the reported numbers about T2D (and rising obesity) that it can feel that we are becoming resistant to an appropriate, more urgent response.

Many people, including doctors, feel intuitively that we now 'overindulge' and don't take good care of ourselves – that we ourselves are to blame. However, modern lifestyles are complex and challenging, and the food environment clearly makes staying healthy difficult. One of the main messages in this book, we hope, is that we have not been in full control of our food choices in particular, which have been driven during this period by a combination of politics, medicine and the food industry. T2D is most definitely our problem, but not, it seems, necessarily our fault.

Something happened around 1980, at least somewhere around that year. We don't mean just that hair got shorter and popular music became 'electronic' – our species started to physically change. We can see that from our T2D graph. Body weight was changing by 1980, though it might have taken another decade for alarm bells to sound. Look at archive photographs, maybe your own, and compare people of the 1970s with those in 2020. In less than two generations – what happened?

Figure 1.4: Rising weight

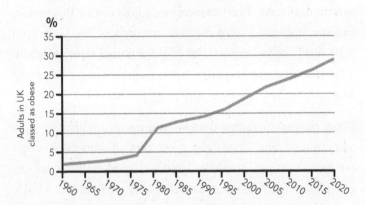

All countries show rises in T2D and weight in the last forty years or so, but the variation is wide. Some have seen a modest increase in average weight but a big rise in T2D, and others the opposite – a bigger rise in weight and a smaller rise in T2D.

Big variations between weight and T2D growth around the world suggest that although being overweight links with T2D, it cannot be a *direct* cause; in any event, at least 15 per cent of people with T2D are lean like Cassie. There are also many very obese people who do not have – and probably will never get – T2D.

Weight gain on its own cannot explain the global pandemic of T2D

We now know that changes in weight and T2D in populations are seeded in the same soil, but they are not the same plant

– and their paths are growing apart. Some of us are susceptible to becoming overweight and some are destined to be at risk from T2D. What drives becoming overweight can drive T2D too, but neither is inevitable, if we can find the safe nutritional path. This is good news – it gives us something to work on, as we cannot change our genes!

Overall, about one in three people in the world is overweight (BMI >25), but in some countries one in three people, or even more, is actually obese (BMI>30). BMI (body mass index) is explained in Appendix 2: Terminology.

People just about everywhere are getting heavier on average – we've all noticed how clothing manufacturers have adapted their sizes – and, worryingly, children are quickly catching up. According to the World Health Organization (WHO), world-wide more than one in five children and young people aged between five and nineteen are overweight. In some countries, such as the US and the UK, around one in five children are actually classed as obese. Even more concerning is that these figures are *still* rising.

Rising weight in children should be a major wake-up call for everyone. Children are programmed to grow, mainly by lengthening rather than fattening, and overweight children often turn into overweight adults, with all of the consequences of that. The rise in T2D will just keep accelerating if the current childhood obesity pandemic is not addressed.

There are more people now with too much energy stored in their bodies than too little. Both are forms of malnutrition.

Liver disease – the rise and rise of NAFLD

Non-alcoholic fatty liver disease, or NAFLD (most folk say 'naff-led') was on very few radars until about 1980. A liver disease, unconnected with either alcohol or infection, emerged after doctors started to see increasing numbers of abnormal liver function blood tests – up to around a quarter of routine tests during the 1990s.

Liver scans of those with abnormal tests nearly always showed a single abnormality – the presence of excess fat. Initially regarded as a harmless manifestation of fat generally, over time we started to see inflammation of the liver, even cirrhosis (scarring of the liver caused by long-term liver damage), as with alcohol. It was most definitely not harmless. We then learned that NAFLD was more common in people with T2D, and people affected by NAFLD were more prone to the same artery diseases as people with T2D. As you will see shortly, excess liver fat is one of the clearest markers of metabolism under stress. Excess liver fat is present in T2D, and both NAFLD and T2D get better if we can eat in a way that helps to clear that fat.

Of our cases, Suzanne, Cassie and Colin all had abnormal liver tests, which became normal when their diets were changed. A diagnosis of 'fatty liver' (as with Alan) means that your liver is making or storing (or both) too much fat, and your body overall is storing too much energy. Excess liver fat impedes the action of insulin – a key step in how T2D starts (see the next chapter).

NAFLD has become the most common liver disease globally,

and appeared at roughly the same time as the escalations in obesity and T2D around 1980. Science can now better explain just how connected these things are.

Insulin resistance and weight gain

This expanding family of conditions also includes high blood pressure and high blood triglyceride (fat) levels, both of which are seen in T2D. It is called metabolic syndrome – metabolic meaning to do with metabolism or energy, and syndrome meaning things which occur together. Metabolic syndrome conditions share the common thread of insulin resistance. The simplest visible clue to its presence is fat around the tummy, which can signal fat *inside* the abdomen or, worse, inside organs like the liver.

When we gain weight, accumulated fat is mainly generalised – spread around the outside of the body under the skin (subcutaneous fat). You can see it and you can feel it! This is the normal and healthy way to store spare energy. Excess fat in organs like the liver is not normal or healthy, and is a major contributor to insulin resistance, and to diseases like T2D.

Nowadays, it's said that on average adults are gaining half a kilogram (just over one pound) every year from the age of twenty onwards. It seems likely that the weight we gain *as an individual* over a period of years contributes to our risk of getting T2D, especially if we have the 'wrong' genes. If you have gained at this rate or more and do not have T2D, it might still show up in the future, or you may be fortunate and are not at risk. If you have good fat storage capacity under the skin, little liver fat and are not susceptible to T2D, you could gain, in theory, a huge amount of weight and stay healthy – think of a sumo wrestler!

To date, we don't have any easy way of knowing our safe fat storage capacity, nor our true genetic predisposition for T2D, so avoiding weight gain is the safe option.

Table 1.1: Previous weight gains over an estimated timescale of our case examples at the time they were diagnosed (TBW = total body weight)

	Weight gain in kg (pounds)	Change in BMI	Timescale of weight gain in years	Increase in TBW (%)
Ted	12 (26)	25–29	40+	16
Cassie	8 (18)	17–20	4	15
Suzanne	13 (29)	24–29	11	20
Mustafa	14 (31)	25–29	6	18
Margaret	15 (33)	25–30	30+	20
Benjamin	16 (35)	30–34	20+	18
Nandita	14 (31)	27–32	25	18
Colin	13 (29)	25–28	30+	15

Their actual weight gains were fairly similar apart from Cassie's, although her percentage weight gain was similar. BMI increases of 3–5 were seen across all cases. It's worth noting that Cassie's weight gain was the smallest, occurred over the shortest time, and she was the most unwell.

EXERCISE

Have you gained weight? If so, how much, and over what timescale?

See if you can pull together a sense of how your weight might have changed over the years. What was your recollection of your weight aged around twenty? Then go up by the decades, using life events, like weddings, births or big holidays (or look at photos) to jog your memory.

Gaining 10–15 per cent of your total body weight, or 10–15kg (20–30lb+ or more) – which can be more than 15 per cent – is quite significant. If you have T2D, a weight loss of the same may be enough to get you started on the road to recovery (see Chapter 5).

Final thoughts on the 1980s

Changes in eating patterns across many countries started in the 1970s when concerns around cholesterol and dietary fat started to make their impact. Comprehensive dietary guidelines – a new departure for governments – appeared in the US in 1977, and in Europe a few years later. This nutritional advice almost certainly accelerated the reduction in dietary fat, which was already under way, with a consequent increase in average carbohydrate intake. Many experts believe that further rises in weight and T2D were linked to these dietary changes, with slowly rising insulin levels being the main driver. The 1980s brought rising weight, T2D, NAFLD and metabolic syndrome.

Before we leave this opening chapter, we want to say a little more about the experience of T2D and what we believe most people need to tackle the disease. We will do that with Cassie, Margaret and Colin, comparing and contrasting their reactions and how they started out.

Cassie

Cassie was super fit and a keen runner for twenty years. At the age of fifty-three, she began to feel unusually tired and running became hard work. She started to get irritating infections and soreness in the skin around her toenails after running. She began to pee a lot and, thinking she had cystitis, made several unproductive visits to the pharmacist. Her energy finally 'switched off' and she had to stop running. She had never been 'properly' ill, so just what was wrong with her? Cancer was on her mind.

What was wrong with her was that she had T2D with a HbA1c of 104mmol/mol or 11.7% (normal <42/6.0%), and her blood glucose level was three times its normal value. There were problems too with her liver blood tests and blood pressure.

Cassie was dumbfounded by the diagnosis of T2D which had not crossed her mind for a moment. How could this have happened to someone as fit as she had been? She felt sad for what had happened to the body she thought she had looked after so well, now broken seemingly for good.

She felt angry at the world, including her friends, some of whom smoked or drank to excess. She thought to herself, Why me? After some very difficult early days, Cassie read that it might be possible to reverse T2D and maybe get her life back again. The start of her fightback was simply that knowledge – it triggered her determination to find a way back to health. Those who knew her would say, 'If anyone can do it, Cassie can.' The determination which drove her to run would now be harnessed to making her well again.

Margaret

Margaret was surprised and disappointed to be diagnosed with T2D, but in truth not shocked. She had always been in good health, but her work as a carer meant that she had seen many people with T2D, and she had an elderly aunt with the disease who seemed to manage well. It felt to her that it was one of those things that people got – a person was lucky not to have it at her age! She knew that her weight needed to be tackled and if she had to take medication then so be it. People would help, and she would do as the doctor and nurse advised.

Margaret was the hub of her family, and did so much for other people that she had rarely thought of doing things for herself.

The nurse advising her about eating well and looking after herself was the first time she had really thought about her health since she was last pregnant over thirty years before! Margaret's best friend had nagged her constantly to go to an exercise class with her at the local leisure centre, and she'd always said she hadn't the time, but maybe she should make time now. It's never too late to get a bit fitter and, after all, she was only sixty-two. She wanted to stay fit for her grandchildren and needed to work for a few more years for the family finances.

Margaret had a sunny disposition which gave no room for glum thoughts, and this would prove invaluable to her in the months and years ahead. She would do well with her T2D but not without some twists and turns, which started not long after she was diagnosed when, sadly, her aunt had a stroke and needed to go into care.

Colin

Colin had such a difficult start to T2D, diagnosed in the immediate aftermath of a heart attack. At the time, it had felt to him like rubbing salt into a wound. It was only much later when he understood that his heart attack had not caused any serious or lasting damage and life had started to look up, that he realised that maybe the heart problem had been a blessing in disguise; he reasoned that it gave him the chance to get control of his T2D before something worse happened.

At the time he was diagnosed, Colin had been depressed for months. His life had been on hold for some time, a redundancy threatened, and he could see no way at his age that he would be able to find another job that paid a decent wage. He had lost interest in everything, rarely went out and was seeing less of his friends. His wife tried hard to galvanise him, but to no avail. If he lost his job, he felt that life would not be worth living.

Colin's depression had taken over his life. The heart attack and T2D together had pushed him even lower, if that were possible. He simply could not take it all in. He had lost all his drive. His wife had to work very hard to get him to see his doctor.

Colin could not engage with his new physical health problems – that would have to be done by his wife and his healthcare team. He received psychological help for his depression, and in time was able to take over control of his T2D, which he came to understand also helped, in turn, his heart and his mood.

The toolkit

Every job has its toolkit, and looking after T2D is no exception. Now that you have a little knowledge – and there is much to come – you can start to think about what *you* need to know or do, and share that with a partner or friend *and* your nurse or doctor. Some of us can do lots for ourselves and some of us need more help, but that's OK and we can all get to the same place eventually. Here are our ideas of what might be in a T2D toolkit, and you can think of your own additions.

Knowledge – you have opened this book and there are many other ways to get knowledge that we'll signpost for you.

Knowledge helps us to understand things, to predict or answer our questions, and can focus our whole approach and trigger us into action. It is important to know that you can, with guidance, put T2D into remission by changing the way you eat, and that medical treatment can help too, though that can't get rid of the T2D itself. Knowledge also helps you to keep a sense of perspective – this is a serious disease but there are worse, and you *can* live well with it.

People help – those attempting to reverse and hold T2D in remission have emphasised the importance of ongoing support from people around them: their healthcare team and, especially, their friends and family. T2D can be a complex experience and your care team will ideally have a diabetes-trained professional who can provide up-to-date technical care but also *personal* continuity of care. Working with professionals who come to know you as a person enables the shared decision-making which is the heart of good care.

Taking control – ideally with a long-term health condition, try to be in charge; what you do yourself will have much more impact than things that medical people do. Believe that. Don't be afraid to experiment – safely. Be guided by what you read but also by your healthcare team. T2D is impacted differently by different approaches in different people; this is especially true for how you eat. Go with what works rather than what should work!

Persistence – keep going! Even if you do perfect self-help, receive perfect healthcare and hit the perfect dietary notes with T2D, it can take a long time to get better. It took Cassie almost a year to feel anywhere near normal, and that was just the beginning. Staying well is a lifelong task but doable. The rewards are definitely worth the effort!

Mindset – is something that could describe us, or part of us, as we can have more than one. It's about attitude and can determine how we approach something and our disposition to act (or not). Being open-minded and wanting to learn is one kind of mindset. Determination and wanting to stay in control of your health are others, and all are really helpful when dealing with T2D.

Motivation – underpinning a determined mindset is motivation, one of the cornerstones of self-help. It's fundamentally how we encourage ourselves to achieve things – to make changes like living healthily. In T2D, lifestyle changes can feel tough, and tougher still to maintain. At times, even the most determined mindset can need refuelling. A person's deepest innermost motivation can provide that fuel. Margaret, for example, felt motivated to stay as healthy as possible, to see her grandchildren grow up.

Pause for thought

If you have recently been diagnosed with T2D, what would you like to happen next (other than a magic spell to remove it!)? What motivates you to change? What else might you need in your toolkit?

Mental health – it can be tricky, if not downright impossible, to manage T2D well with a significant mental health issue hovering. Mental health problems nearly always need to be tackled first, while 'holding' T2D as safely as possible, which is what happened with Colin. They are both common and will often overlap. The challenge of managing them both will be looked at later in the book. Our minds are intertwined with our bodies so it is not possible to receive a life-changing diagnosis without there being an emotional reaction.

This does not mean that you also now have a diagnosis of a mental health problem, but it is normal to feel a range of emotions – from sadness, anger and anxiety to difficulty accepting the diagnosis. Depression and anxiety are common in people with T2D and should not be ignored. There may be a sense of grief about aspects of life that seem lost. Typical thoughts can be: 'It's not fair.' 'Why do bad things always happen to me?' 'My life can never be as good again.' 'It's all my fault.' 'I should have been able to stop this from happening', etc. These experiences are completely normal. In Chapters 10 and 11, we will consider ways of looking after your mental wellbeing when you are adjusting to the diagnosis and also for along the way when things don't go to plan, and how to pick yourself up again. We'll look at ways you can help yourself and also ways of accessing help if needed.

Pause for thought

What was the main emotion you felt when you were diagnosed with T2D? What thoughts went through your mind? Do you still experience the same emotions and thoughts? If not, how have they changed?

Introducing FAST

When a person fasts, they stop eating for a certain period of time. Fasting is generally a healthy thing to do and can be very helpful in T2D; we are going to talk about fasting in the food chapters, 5 and 6. We would like to introduce you now to another kind of fast – one using each letter of the word to make a T2D health check reminder:

FAST stands for **F**ood, **A**ctivity, **S**leep, **T**ension. By activity we also mean exercise, and by tension we mean persisting stress or worry of any kind. We judged FAST to be easier and more useful than FESS!

You have four prongs on your weapon or, if you prefer, four routes of attack to hit back at T2D: eating as well as you can; being as active as possible; getting your best sleep; dealing with your stresses and tensions to the best of your ability. It's likely that the cause of your T2D lies within these areas – it might be one or more – so addressing them all gives you the best chance of putting your T2D right, or at least of making things a good deal better.

Though we will refer to F-A-S-T throughout the book, the F chapters are 5 and 6, the A chapter is 3, the S chapter is 4, and the T chapters are 10 and 11. You can think about FAST at every annual or anniversary T2D check-up or every clinic check with your diabetes healthcare team; once a month, every week or even every day, just in your own way! Use it as you go, or when a problem arises, or when managing T2D gets tough, which happens.

It's a quick and easy reminder that four things matter with T2D – not just one. You can think about FAST as often or as seldom as you like – or use something similar of your own creation – whatever works for you.

Key points from Chapter 1

- T2D comes on slowly, possibly over years, and presents in a variety of ways. Most people don't feel especially ill early on.

- An elevated blood glucose level (hyperglycaemia) is only a part of T2D.

- A diagnosis of T2D can be based on a raised glucose (fasting blood sample) or raised HbA1c test. The tests are related but not the same.

- T2D is significantly different to T1D and are not connected in the same person – you don't get both!

- Weight gain and insulin resistance are the hallmarks of T2D.

- Some 15 per cent or more of people with T2D are of normal weight (lean).

- Average weight and T2D have risen dramatically during the last forty years or so.

- T2D is part of a metabolic syndrome of related conditions, which also includes fatty liver disease (NAFLD) and high blood pressure (hypertension).

- T2D is not 'mild' diabetes.

- A diagnosis of T2D can provoke a wide variety of emotional, but mainly normal, responses.

- FAST is a reminder to think widely about the causes of T2D, and the ways to address it.

Metabolism: the basics, and what happens in type 2 diabetes

If you are familiar with basic nutrition terms and know what carbohydrates (including sugars), fats and proteins are, then read on. If not, there is an option to look at a short explanation in Appendix 2: Terminology (for Chapter 2).

What exactly is metabolism? Clearly from conversations it means slightly different things to different people:

- 'Is it to do with digestion?'

- 'It's to do with our weight, I think.'

- 'Something to do with food and vitamins?'

- 'I have a thyroid problem which slowed down my metabolism.'

- 'I feel so tired, so it must be to do with energy.'

These were a few comments from people we asked, and they are all partly right. How might you describe metabolism? A scientist might say that it is the sum total of the things that go on in the cells of our body to keep everything working and to keep us alive. In other words, metabolism is life – it's why we are not rocks!

A human body has lots of systems, all interconnected to keep us alive and healthy. You will be relieved to know that we are only going to focus on one system here – the part of metabolism that involves energy balance in the body, and especially the way that our body uses its two main fuels – glucose and fat. The body's energy system is so central to life that scientists and doctors have come to use 'metabolic' to mean things to do with fuel (food) and energy. Things that go wrong with this system are called metabolic problems or diseases. T2D is a metabolic disease because problems with insulin radically affect the way our body stores and uses energy.

In fact, T2D is the most typical metabolic disease. The body's systems control how we grow, how we reproduce, how we use energy, how we move, how we repair damage, contain illness and so forth, and in the brain, we have a system for managing the systems.

They are all very complex – beyond complex almost – but they all seem to follow some simple rules:

Things are kept constant, steady and safe. You might recognise the word **homeostasis** (see Figure 2.1). It's about how the body will work, sometimes battle, to keep things constant. Living systems remain surprisingly ordered, which is lucky for their owners! Homeostasis looks after us.

Figure 2.1: Homeostasis

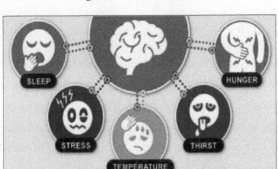

Gordon, L. and Levkowitz, G. (2021)

Homeostasis is the constant conversation between the brain and the rest of the body to keep our physical condition steady and balanced. All the body's systems are joined up – for example, we can easily sense how hunger connects with sleep and stress.

Systems are linked together – though that might not seem very obvious. They are strongly interwoven. Our energy-balance system sits somewhere in the middle. It's central to human life – a bit like the engine and fuel in a car – and without it everything else stops. If we don't get enough energy or can't use it well, we can't grow or reproduce efficiently – we get tired, and moving is difficult; fighting infections is difficult when energy is in short supply. We observed the difficulties people with T2D experienced during the height of the COVID-19 pandemic. More understanding of these elaborate links is shaping our view of how things work.

Finally, systems, messaging and our whole human self are controlled by a super-management system of unfathomable complexity called the brain. Every one of us has a brain (though sometimes those close to us may wonder!) which supervises, monitors, adjusts and readjusts all the other systems so that they are kept steady and work well.

Energy and the brain

The brain is doing a lot more than most of us think to regulate when and what we eat, and how much and what type of fuel goes where in the body. We are more or less oblivious to these regulating functions of our brain. Basic signals, such as hunger and fullness, or satiety, are simply the conscious tip of an iceberg of subconscious brain activity and signalling that keep metabolism working. We don't control the signals; we don't choose to be hungry after exercise, we don't choose to feel lethargic when we are dieting and we don't choose to have a sweet tooth! We can choose or learn how to react to the signals – but we don't *knowingly* put them there.

Hunger is nature's way of telling us that we need some fuel. Lethargy or fatigue is what we feel when the brain is making the body divert energy. For example, if we cut our energy intake (such as when we go on a diet to lose weight) the body detects the fuel cut and reduces the energy it spends internally to protect its fuel store. As a result, we get lethargic and feel cold. Weight loss is understandably hard when the body is naturally trying to do the opposite! The sweet tooth is harder to explain but might become clearer later.

When the control mechanisms for energy balance are faulty – and they definitely are in T2D – there is a breakdown in some very basic mechanisms. Hunger is a good example of 'signalling' gone wrong. In health, hunger is there just when we need it. But in T2D most people complain of always or often feeling hungry – yet the body is literally overflowing with energy. Why does that happen? Why would a power station manager send for more coal when all his storage is full, and why does a person with T2D – with a body full of stored energy – send for more? Read on!

Energy metabolism – the basics

So, what do we need, and what has to happen to keep us alive and well?

Just like a car (again), we need **air**, **water** and **fuel**. It's easy to think that all we need for healthy metabolism is fuel for our 'engine', but air and water are also essential – we breathe and drink because both have a big role in making and managing energy too.

Air (oxygen) – There's a reason for life starting on a planet with some oxygen in the atmosphere: it's one of a small number of key elements needed for life and is so important that, if we go more than a few minutes without it, we die. It's vital to most of the chemistry in our cells, especially those in the brain. When the fuel in our food – that's fat and glucose – is 'burned', it reacts with oxygen and that reaction releases energy.

FOOD + OXYGEN → ENERGY to: - Move and think

- Stay warm, keep alert

- Stay alive

To stay alive, we need the energy to fuel all our unseen 'background' systems which run our body, rather like the autopilot on an aeroplane. Energy we are conscious of using – including exercise – makes up about a third of what we use, and the rest (most of it) feeds the autopilot.

Water – As with oxygen, life could not have started on Earth without water. Scientists say that if you want to find life on other planets, look for water. We can struggle through a few days without drinking water, but not much more. Most of our body is water; it helps us to keep the concentration of chemicals in our cells at precisely the right level for correct functioning and helps us to get rid of anything surplus to requirements. Water plays a big part in energy metabolism, too.

You may have wondered what happens to your surplus fat if you do manage to shed some excess weight. After taking the energy from the fat molecules, our bodies turn what's left into carbon dioxide and water, and we literally breathe and pee it all away! Water is *in* our food, but we also *make* it from food.

Fat + oxygen → energy + carbon dioxide + water

Fuel – The bulk of our food is composed of carbohydrates, fats and protein, and 80–85 per cent of our daily energy needs are met by carbohydrates (as glucose) and fats (as fatty acids).

These are the body's two primary fuels. What we actually use depends on our diet, but overall a half or more of most people's daily food energy comes from glucose, about 30 per cent from fat, with around 15 per cent from protein. Fat and glucose are to the body what petrol and diesel have been to cars, but the body, being able to switch easily from one to the other, is more like a modern hybrid car.

Proteins – These are incredibly special and important to life and to overall metabolism, but in energy terms their contribution is relatively small. We might think we all need more protein for vitality, but the body knows what it needs and anything in excess it turns into other forms of energy – including fat. It's easy to gain around the middle rather than in the muscles when using protein shakes!

Fuel on the go

Glucose – This is on hand in the bloodstream 24/7, to be delivered to any part of the body – to any cell wherever and whenever needed. We intuitively connect glucose with energy, and energy with movement, but as we just said, most of our daily energy goes not on moving our body but on the internal systems which together keep us alive and well. Not surprisingly, the organ that directs those systems, the brain, takes the lion's share of that background energy – about a third in fact – all to itself!

Think too of the energy needed to make our second most important organ – the heart – beat around a hundred thousand times a day. Just being alive and not moving takes a lot of energy! So each of us spends about a third of our energy doing 'stuff' – walking, talking, working, etc. We also keep a little more for unexpected bursts of activity, such as running for a bus or away from danger. This is triggered by a release of adrenaline, leading to the extra surge of glucose needed for the muscle work to catch the bus or escape the charging bull.

The amount of glucose in the bloodstream at any one time is remarkably small – little more than a teaspoonful. Not much fuel to look after a fully grown human, you might think! So clearly, we need a mechanism for keeping that glucose level continuously topped up, so that energy is always on hand. Glucose in the bloodstream also needs to be kept stable. Too little glucose and cells can be starved of energy – the brain being particularly sensitive. A drop to less than half the normal level can cause coma, but too much can damage blood vessels, as happens in all forms of diabetes.

The controls on this system work well in a healthy person, but when things go wrong, as happens in T2D, some of those protections are lost and glucose can get too high at any time, but especially after eating. So keeping glucose at the right level is essential and when we are healthy, all works well.

Fat – As will already be obvious to you, fat is different to glucose. However, as we've seen, the body can run on both fuels. Generally, about a third of our energy needs are met by fat, although it varies quite a bit from person to person. Fat is a less speedy fuel than glucose – it's slower to kick in – so it's not normally the fuel used to run away from bulls! However, it is remarkably flexible, and although in most people it provides the bulk of stored energy for use later rather than now, it can, with suitable lifestyle adjustments, replace glucose as the main go-to fuel with surprising ease.

We think of fat as a back-up fuel, but some organs use it as a daily first choice over glucose. Heart muscle cells take most of their energy from the fatty acids in fat, which is ironic in view of our recent association of fat with heart disease!

After eating and digestion, fat moves from the intestine into the general circulation and fat stores, bypassing the main depot of the liver where everything else, notably glucose, is heading. There is always fat in the bloodstream, on its way between the intestine, fat stores and the liver, and it can be used to supply cells, such as muscles, with energy. Unlike glucose, the level of fat in the bloodstream has no effect on the way we feel.

So fat regulation is less strict than glucose; it tends to be a back-up and storage fuel, but can be used in the moment (the heart), and can take over the lead provider role for the body generally if needed.

Staying alive is a complicated business under the surface. We use energy constantly – whether we are active or not – but we are evolved to eat at intervals for all sorts of (mainly obvious) reasons. Sometimes we don't eat at all for a day or longer, and every day we don't eat when we sleep. So we have always needed a fuel and engine management system that allows for variations in food intake. Energy, in the moment, *has* to come from some place other than food directly!

Stored fuel

Still sticking with our two main fuels, let's see how the body solves its energy storage problem.

Glucose can be stored. In plants we call it starch, and it's mainly in roots and seeds. The thickened underground stems of plants like potatoes – the tubers – are full of starch to feed the plant and to feed *us* when we make chips! In animals, like us humans, the equivalent of starch is glycogen, which is many thousands of glucose molecules joined together. Glycogen is mainly a muscle fuel, with a smaller back-up store in the liver. Glycogen stores are not big – about 2000kcal in total – enough to fuel the body on a lazy day but not much more! We can't store a lot of energy as glucose/glycogen as it requires a bulky water 'jacket' which limited body space prevents!

Glycogen is quickly available but doesn't last long. If day-to-day energy use is like having money in your pocket, glycogen gives you the comfort of a few notes – you could cover an unexpected visit to a bar or restaurant for example, but to buy a big item, you'd need your bank card – and that's fat!

Fat is the opposite of glucose as a storage material, and an example of why we have evolved to use both, as they do complement each other. Fat is the optimum storage material; it takes up less space in the body relative to the amount of energy it holds (a lot!) and can be broken down quite quickly under the right conditions.

Small amounts of fat can be stored in our cells as tiny fat

droplets – a rapid energy source. In people who are more adapted to burning fat rather than glucose, such as some athletes, the number and size of fat droplets increases, and this is a normal and healthy part of metabolism.

The bigger, more familiar storage site for fat, under our skin, our subcutaneous fat, provides us with both padding and insulation but in energy terms is truly a marvel of evolutionary engineering and plays a big role in keeping us alive! We can survive two or three months of starvation on average body fat stores – women longer than men.

Manufactured fuel

Not only do we eat and store fuel, but we *make* it! In balancing energy in the body, moment-to-moment, we juggle with three balls – healthy metabolism is the interplay between eating, storing and making fuel.

Making fuel is about swapping things around and our brilliant liver allows us to make most things from just about most other things.

What you eat will dictate how much of your food fuel will cover your **glucose** energy needs. Glycogen can cover short gaps and unexpected surges – but most of the glucose we use is actually *made* in the liver.

Making glucose is one of the most important things the liver does, ensuring that it's always around, especially for the brain, which is glucose-needy and is always first in the queue for fuel!

About a quarter of all the energy used by the body each day is used by the brain, so the demand for glucose is always there. The supply tap of glucose from the liver is more or less set in the 'on' position, and only gets turned down/off after meals, when glucose floods in from digestion of food. So when we eat carbohydrates, glucose is available from food and less needs to be made by the liver. When we eat fewer carbohydrates, the liver takes over and makes whatever we need!

Fat in both our food and in stores can usually be used for energy. But we also make fat, and this is done mainly within the fat tissue store itself, and more importantly, from a T2D angle, we make fat in the liver, and we'll see why this matters shortly.

When the supply of glucose is plentiful (carbohydrate-rich food), and the 'piggy bank' of glycogen is full, any excess glucose is turned into fat by the liver and moved on into fat tissue for storage. This is good, normal metabolism – we might not like the 'love handles' but it's how nature works and causes no harm.

Using energy to power up the body is a balancing act between glucose and fat, and it's all decided by the brain and liver – these organs work out for us what needs to be done, leaving us to get on with our day!

In relation to our main fuels, the liver is a depot, factory and distribution centre for both fat and glucose – it is the fuel hub of the body.

Insulin is made and released by the pancreas (Figure 2.2), which sits below and behind the stomach, and is joined up along with the liver to the upper part of the intestine. This area is where nearly all the main digestive action takes place. The pancreas nestles into a bend in the small intestine into which it releases digestive juices, along with those from the gallbladder.

The liver has, uniquely, two blood supplies: one from the general circulation, like all other organs, and another branch line or 'fast track' blood supply from the intestine and digestion. Its purpose is to take the products of digestion (from carbohydrates and proteins) directly to the liver. This fast-track blood vessel is called the portal vein.

The pancreas, apart from supplying digestive juices into the small intestine, manufactures insulin which is released into the portal vein, reaching the liver directly and quickly.

Figure 2.2: The upper digestive system – viewed from the front

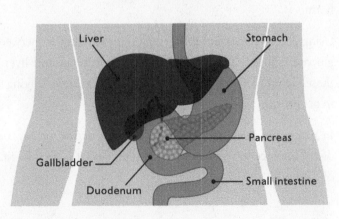

Fat from digestion leaves the intestine by a completely different route, as its packaging would not fit into the tiny blood
vessels that allow all other nutrients to pass into the fast-track
vessel to the liver. Fat digestion contributes little, if anything,
to insulin release. It's useful to recall this when thinking later
about eating to keep insulin levels lower – and if you are on
insulin, it's one of the reasons why a fattier meal requires
much less insulin to manage the fuel coming into the liver
after eating.

Insulin and food

Before food is eaten, during a meal and for an hour or two
afterwards, insulin is on the go, and its job is to meet and greet
the incoming wave of fuel. After digestion, it directs the fuel
into the appropriate channels, like a traffic cop. Let's look at
what happens when we eat spaghetti bolognese.

Firstly, the smell of food triggers digestive juices and gets
insulin ready for work. During digestion, the pasta releases
its carbohydrate as glucose, along with a little more from the
sauce, which, after absorption into the bloodstream, triggers
the release of insulin, as does protein, mainly from the sauce
(meat or not). Fat coming from the sauce does not trigger insulin. Most of the insulin released by eating spaghetti bolognese
is triggered by the pasta.

After the first wave of fuel and insulin are circulating, the
insulin begins its job of allocating the fuel. Glucose in the
bloodstream is transported into cells, and its blood level

drops. Insulin turns down the glucose supply tap at the liver and the blood level drops some more. Both of the main actions of insulin on glucose cause the blood level to go down.

Fat from the bolognese sauce and its contents circulates after digestion and moves into fat stores under the skin, the liver and into cells for later use. Insulin pushes fat into store and locks it in place. Whenever glucose and insulin are around, fat is mainly stored and not used for energy there and then.

Glucose is what we absorb into the bloodstream when carbohydrates are digested – which is most of our bread, rice, pasta, potatoes and much of our fruit. Our pasta meal, with a little bread on the side, is going to come in at around 100g of carbohydrate (therefore glucose) making up around half the calories in this 800kcal dinner.

> **Pause for thought**
>
> Think of your typical main meal. What percentage would you guess is made up of carbohydrates such as bread, rice, pasta, potatoes and fruit?

Spaghetti bolognese, a very typical meal in terms of its nutrients, is going to deliver, within an hour or so, a large 'glug' – 100g (22 teaspoons) – of glucose into the bloodstream which normally contains only 5g (just over one teaspoon). One of the most important actions of insulin is to prevent a tidal wave of glucose flooding the circulation, and we can sense from these numbers how big a problem this would be without a healthy insulin response.

About half of the glucose from our dinner will supply the body's energy needs for a few hours – notably those of the brain. About half – under the guidance of insulin – is put into short-term storage in the liver, and especially the muscles. The glucose production tap at the liver is switched off within about thirty minutes of eating, and the surge of insulin, peaking an hour after eating, has fallen back to its baseline after a further hour.

So, not long after eating, insulin has directed glucose into fuel use or storage and has maintained a safe blood level even when a lot of carbohydrate has been eaten. This dynamic two-hour processing operation occurs, in all healthy people, after each meal, and prevents the very big surge in blood glucose which would happen in the absence of insulin.

Insulin and fat

Insulin is the body's 'squirrel' – it makes us store food energy in any form, and fat is no exception. The fat in our bolognese sauce gets mainly tucked away into temporary storage, and can only be used as fuel when insulin levels drop.

This is because insulin acts like a lock on our fat stores. While insulin is raised in the bloodstream to deal with glucose, fat stores stay tightly shut, so the burning of fat anywhere in the body becomes difficult.

This means that, although we are dual fuel, we tend in any given moment to be burning glucose *or* fat and not both at the same time – a bit like the hybrid car where we're running on liquid fuel or battery at any one time.

Insulin encourages fat storage and hinders its use as a fuel, and in an ironic twist of metabolism, the small size of our glucose (glycogen) stores means that surplus glucose – if we like to eat plenty of pasta – can't be stored as glucose, and the body's only option is to convert it to fat – which the liver does extremely efficiently!

If, day by day, we consume more energy than we can handle, and especially if a sizeable chunk of that energy is glucose, which has limited storage and triggers insulin and fat-storing, then the body is literally in fat-making and storage mode and we gain weight.

Fat storage promoted by insulin has occurred during a period when, ironically, we have eaten less fat but more carbohydrates, certainly more than fifty years ago – and we may be eating them more often (snacking). Both will stimulate more insulin than is really good for us.

EXERCISE

Start thinking about your own snacking

Snacking – also known as 'grazing' – might be an issue for T2D and we'll look at this a bit more in Chapter 6. If you eat between meals, and most of us do, start to think now about your own snacking behaviour. We'll look at monitoring and using diaries later in the book, but a piece of paper and pen are all you need for now. Make a note of when, where and why you were snacking, and what the snack was. Try to do this over a week, updating throughout each day as you go.

Monitoring eating is a big help in managing T2D. At its basic level, it connects you with the reality of what you are doing rather than the optimistic guesswork of memory – and sometimes that connection is enough for us to change the thing that we are monitoring. But this is overweight, not T2D – something else has to happen for T2D to appear on the scene.

Insulin has been rising

Measuring insulin is not usually a routine laboratory test that your doctor can order but researchers have been able to study it for about sixty years, and we know that rising levels of both insulin and glucose have been with us for three or four decades – a timeline matching that of rising obesity and T2D.

On average, glucose is up a little, but insulin much more, which tells us that our pancreas is having to work much harder to keep glucose safe. Some of us are making two, three or even more times as much insulin as people did a few decades ago. Up to a point, our pancreas can manage this – it has a good reserve – and things will still work normally. But to repeat: a higher insulin level, for whatever reason, will cause weight gain. The same happens, unfortunately, when we use insulin to manage blood glucose.

Rising insulin is an exceptional and worrisome change in the way our bodies are working. Like rising global temperatures, it should trigger an alarm response. Why is this happening? And what can we do to stop it? Rising insulin levels are connected to rising weight, and may be a big part of its cause.

Have you ever lived next to a busy road and realised that, over a period of time, the sound of traffic seems less? Or have you been given a clock with a loud tick, which you almost stop noticing after a while? We get used to things – the brain turns down the volume for us to make life more comfortable. We get less sensitive, or more resistant, to something bothersome.

Rising insulin may have caused the body to turn down its insulin volume control, to protect us from the possibility of blood glucose going too low (insulin lowers blood glucose, of course). This makes sense, but being more resistant to insulin naturally triggers more insulin to be made to keep glucose stable and safe. The body appears then to be in a tail-chasing spiral.

The best scientific brains have been pondering for many years why we get the insulin resistance which drives T2D and related conditions. Simply making too much insulin and having too much liver fat are looking like prime suspects.

Insulin resistance is to T2D what absent insulin is to T1D, but because resistance develops over many years, the creep upwards of blood glucose is also over a long time period. At some point, a tipping point occurs, probably triggered by a critical level of excess liver fat, and insulin resistance gets worse more quickly; blood glucose rises sharply, especially after meals, not returning fully to normal levels.

In the early stage, insulin, insulin resistance and glucose, hand in hand, are all going up. Insulin production in the pancreas is in overdrive; this is the high insulin of early T2D.

Figure 2.3: T2D stage 1 – rising insulin

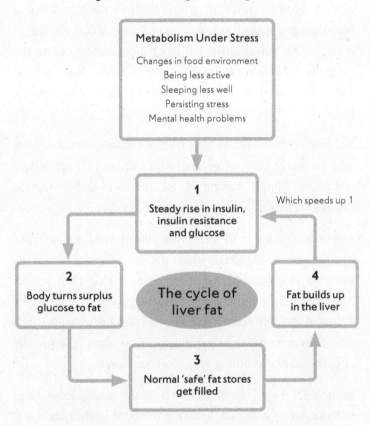

*This cycle builds up over years (or decades) but speeds up
after step 4. Insulin levels are high. Eating too much and/or
the wrong food is likely to be the main problem in most of us;
but lack of exercise, poor sleep and mental health problems all
impact insulin resistance (as discussed in the next two chapters).*

Advancing T2D

Figure 2.4: T2D stage 2 – falling insulin

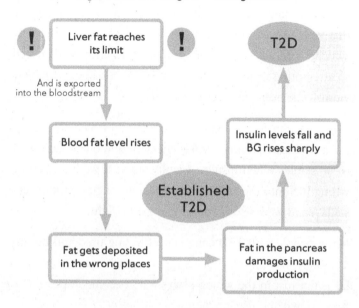

As well as increasing insulin resistance, a fat-overloaded liver will pass some of that fat into the circulation and on into other organs; even a small amount of fat in the pancreas can switch off insulin production. BG = blood glucose.

We think of T2D as being about raised blood glucose, but it is just as much about too much fat, and fat where it is not meant to be.

The timeline for all this could be decades to just three or four years or less, especially so in a slim person with the 'wrong' genes – someone like Cassie. The final phase when fat is coming out of the liver, affecting the pancreas and damaging insulin production, probably occurs over about one or two years. The symptoms of raised blood glucose can appear at any point, and everyone's different. Recent research suggests that cells in the pancreas damaged by deposited fat may be switched off (sleeping) rather than permanently damaged, so attempting to reverse the changes (see Chapter 5) may be worthwhile even after many years of T2D.

When insulin functions well, the engine of metabolism is a quiet well-tuned hum – we feel energetic and our weight tends to be stable. When insulin is faulty, it's as if we have put the wrong fuel into the tank – our metabolic 'engine' stutters and stalls – and we lose our energy and gain weight.

Many people with T2D complain of feeling tired and hungry. The body may have lots of energy on board, but accumulating fat is not just in the wrong places – it's become impossible to break down and use for energy.

The wider effects of insulin resistance

We've been looking at fat and glucose in T2D, but insulin has so many roles in the body, and insulin resistance plays a wider part in the health problems that come with T2D, such as NAFLD and being overweight. All three of these things connect too with a much higher risk of artery disease, which should be our main concern. Insulin resistance is associated with high blood pressure, artery damage and a higher risk of clotting. With T2D, you are more likely to have a stroke, poor limb circulation or a heart attack – like Colin.

In short, artery disease, the disease which kills the most people, may well be driven by insulin malfunctions, which in turn are created by the way we live, especially the way we eat. A popular sound bite is 'heart-healthy food'. It's looking like a more helpful approach would be to think about 'liver-healthy food'. To look after our heart (and circulation) we first need to look after our liver. The current health status of human beings makes disturbing reading:

- Overweight: well over half of us.

- NAFLD: one in four people.

- Artery disease: about one in eight people.

- T2D: around one in fifteen people.

Converging estimates from around the world suggest that as many as one in three of us or more have a degree of insulin resistance, including now younger people and children. Many scientists now think it may have an even wider role, for example in conditions like cancer and dementia. Insulin really is a unique substance and may be even more important than we could have imagined.

We can inherit some insulin resistance, which then makes us more susceptible to T2D. But most experts think that genetics plays a fairly small role in this whole process. Most of it comes down to the way we live. We've talked about insulin resistance and the struggle of energy management we now see in the human body. But what really lies beneath this problem with insulin?

As far as we can tell, metabolic syndrome (including many cancers) is relatively new on an evolutionary scale – if we call it fifty to one hundred years, it is the blink of an eye against the one or two million years or more of human evolution. And T2D is very much a disease of the last few decades. Insightful perspectives on this dramatically changed landscape and the metabolic challenges to modern-day humans can be found in the world of evolutionary biology:

> *'For more than 2.5 million years, our metabolic adaptation to seasonal food availability was considered to be an outstanding survival advantage. Nowadays, the same survival strategy in a completely altered surrounding is responsible for a constant body fat accumulation for periods of food deficiency, which will, however, very likely not appear again.'*
>
> Freese, Klement, et al, 2017

We evolved to cope with changes in food availability and have systems which adapted to allow for both fasting periods and an unpredictable and widely varying diet. Switching between foraged plants, fruits and animal fats was manageable because we can metabolise glucose and fat equally well.

But (for nearly all of us) our primal lifestyle is long gone. The modern food environment is built around the constant availability of energy-dense yet often nutrient-poor foods. Our twin fuel system, with its built-in checks and balances, is being progressively dominated by a single macronutrient – the carbohydrate. Add in concerns over psycho-emotional stress, sleep adequacy and whether we are active enough, and the recipe for metabolic disease starts to unfold. It's tough being a modern human!

The good news is that you don't need to become a hunter-gatherer to avoid or fix insulin resistance; it can be prevented or banished by targeting weight loss sufficiently to significantly reduce liver fat. This can reverse or substantially improve T2D, along with all the conditions which connect, including NAFLD and high blood pressure. The potential health gains for getting this right, therefore, are large for all of us.

Experts all say that the earlier in the process we try to tackle T2D by its roots, the more likely we are to succeed. Attempting reversal, the subject of Chapter 5, is easier in the first decade, preferably within five or six years of diagnosis, but there are reports of people managing this after twenty years, demonstrating that insulin failure is not always permanent.

Because insulin resistance cannot be 'medicated' away, this has to be done naturally. The next four chapters are really about doing just that – first by being more active or exercising more, then by improving sleep if necessary, and finally by tackling eating for T2D – full on!

Key points from Chapter 2

- The body's systems are interconnected and all managed by the brain.

- Our cells use two main fuels – glucose and fat (fatty acids).

- Insulin is the body's key energy manager.

- In T2D, insulin resistance (a malfunction) – rather than missing insulin – is the main feature.

- Problems with insulin in T2D trap the body in an energy storage mode, which worsens hunger, tiredness and weight gain.

- Insulin resistance is strongly linked to having too much insulin and too much liver fat (an issue of food choices).

- Dietary measures to lower insulin production and insulin resistance, and avoid excess liver fat could prevent T2D.

- Cells in the pancreas responsible for insulin may be switched off rather than 'dead' in later T2D, giving hope for recovery from T2D.

Being active for type 2 diabetes: exercising common sense

F<u>A</u>ST – being active or exercising?

Being as active as you can is one of your four main options for standing up to T2D, and we'll explain why and how in this chapter.

The words 'active' and 'exercising' both appear in the title of the chapter because both are in common use, and we ourselves are not sure there is a right or wrong term for just moving more! Most people take 'being active' to describe a lifestyle – moving more in general. This might involve, for example, walking or cycling to work, using stairs in buildings, gardening and doing housework, and keeping physically busy in general. 'Exercise' is more a planned session of activity outside of our regular day-to-day schedule, usually over a set time, and targeting fitness and health. We often expend more effort and energy during exercise but over a shorter time. It's not an either/or thing – some people do both.

But being active is how we evolved to be. Looking back in time at our evolutionary past gives a clearer view of the difference between exercising and being active. Humans have been around for over two million years, and our own species, Homo sapiens, for at least two hundred thousand years. For almost all of that time, until agriculture and permanent settlements appeared about twelve thousand years ago, humans hunted and gathered food, leading a nomadic existence. Scientific studies can confirm what you might think would be obvious: that our early ancestors were very active by current standards. Studies of the few surviving hunter-gatherer populations show that much of their day is spent moving, mainly walking. Though widely variable, distances covered can average up to 8 miles (13km) for men and 5 miles (8km) for women. Only small amounts of time are spent doing what in a gym would be called vigorous, but activity is needed every single day – no lazy Sundays!

For 99 per cent of our historic timeline, humans had to be active to survive, and our systems and behaviours became hardwired around that necessity. The concept of exercise for health, or to burn off excess energy and lose weight, would make no sense to a hunter-gatherer. When not in pursuit of food, the Hadza of northern Tanzania – one of the most studied of surviving hunter-gatherer populations – spend their time being sedentary. However, even their version of being still is more active than ours; sitting is unusual except on the floor, and both kneeling and squatting are commonly employed. Along with performing sedentary chores back at base, and without chairs, they are still engaging their muscles more than you might think.

Agriculture changed the world for ever. Wandering for most people stopped, though life remained physically challenging. Being active as farm labourers meant people worked even harder for a living than their nomadic forbears. Then during the last few thousand years, as the first kingdoms and empires developed, we saw the beginning of sports and exercise for military purposes. It seems that nearly all human cultures have embraced sport as a kind of purposeful play into adulthood.

> *'Eating alone will not keep a man well, he must also take exercise . . . And it is necessary, as it appears, to discern the power of various exercises, both natural exercises and artificial.'*
>
> Hippocrates, *Regimen*, circa 400 BC

Hippocrates, revered by many as the father of modern medicine, is credited as the first physician to believe that disease was a product of environmental factors – not ill-fortune or the gods. He clearly grasped the importance of both being active and exercise. He also said, 'Food and exercise, while possessing opposite qualities, yet work together to produce health', and with remarkable foresight, that food can 'overpower exercise'. A point that many of us are currently trying to make!

Over two thousand years later, the Industrial Revolution began by degrees to make life less physically demanding, but advanced mechanisation in the most recent decades has made being active not just unnecessary but actually more difficult for many people.

If the Homo sapiens timeline were an imaginary working day, starting at 9 a.m. and finishing at 5 p.m., we would be hunter-gathering until about 4.45 p.m. Farming and civilisations would fit into the last fifteen minutes and advanced mechanisation would be a matter of seconds. The evolution of our physiology occurred over a very long time frame; how we now live, which has changed over a very short time frame, must be viewed against the many millennia which forged that physiology.

So why do *we* need to be active or exercise at all? Unsurprisingly given our heritage, good health appears to be dependent, in part, on not being completely sedentary. In the last fifty or so years, we have observed and scientifically connected changes in human society and our lifestyles with the sharp rise in metabolic diseases like T2D, high blood pressure and artery disease. Though it is always difficult to tease out the influence of one factor from others that can impact on disease, we can be absolutely confident that if we are less active, we are more susceptible to disease, whether it be physical or psychological. Our chemistry changes adversely if we are not active – or perhaps more accurately we lack the beneficial changes that being active (or exercising) brings.

We have evolved to be active, not to exercise, but exercise is now becoming the main way to maintain that active heritage for many of us. Yet doing something unnatural can feel hard sometimes, especially on the occasions that we just don't feel like doing it. We also need to be kind to ourselves if our bodies are not set well to burn energy, as can be the case if you have been overweight and inactive for a while. Achieving some dietary weight loss first, before trying to step up exercise, is usually helpful.

It's also worth bearing in mind that the transition from being active to exercising is something of a grey zone. Very recent research shows that small health gains can accumulate from even minor adjustments in our daily routines. We can still be more active in the era of exercise; merging the two is good for us, as Hippocrates might have been suggesting.

In recent times, the concept of exercise has been medicalised, politicised and commercialised. At the beginning of the 1980s, US newspapers talked about the 'fitness craze' of exercise, which had gathered up about half of the American adult population. This explosion of recreational exercise came from the conviction of nutritionists in the US that exercise was a guaranteed way to lose weight and become healthier. We needed to respond in particular to the steady reduction of physical activity in the workplace, and to the increasing use of motorised transport. Public health initiatives on exercise followed in the footsteps of earlier nutritional advice, and the modern public health message (adapted by politicians) of 'move more, eat less' was born. We were advised to walk, jog or cycle (or any other way to break sweat) three or four times a week. This kick-started a new health and fitness industry, and gyms or 'fitness centres' began to spring up in towns and cities around the world. If you are over sixty you might remember this happening – parks did not always have joggers!

What does exercise do for health – especially for T2D?

Exercise, as you will see shortly, produces an impressive list of health benefits and is available to most of us – often free of charge! Some of the gains are well known, and to most of us have become beliefs, but they are also generally supported by science and research. The most important ones are:

Exercise improves metabolism. It lowers blood pressure overall, lowers the risk of artery disease, NAFLD and T2D, and we tend to live longer as a result. It also appears to have a favourable effect on cancer risk and dementia.

Research suggests that we can reduce our risk of developing T2D by as much as 25 per cent by being moderately active for half an hour five times a week, and by a third if we double that to five hours a week. Two hours a day could cut your risk in half, though that seems extreme; most of us would struggle with the time commitment unless some of that was covered by just being active, walking or cycling to get around – in which case that massive benefit could be achievable!

- 2.5 hours a week reduces the risk of developing T2D by a quarter.

- 5 hours a week reduces that risk by a third.

- 14 hours a week could cut the risk by 50 per cent!

It's for each person to decide how to play the effort–benefit game – with benefits assumed and into the future, it won't appeal to all – but everyone *feels* better, and that's in the here-and-now!

Exercise improves mental health. It has always been known to benefit people with depression, more than just feeling better immediately afterwards, and is an excellent way of relieving anxiety both in the moment and ongoing if done often enough. The effects on the brain are, not surprisingly, complex. We see favourable effects on stress-linked hormones, on the chemistry of mood, and on the quality of our thinking and processing. The impact of purposeful, sustained exercise can be as much as that from a successful course of antidepressant medication. But then we have all the things that come from socialising and an enhanced sense of self-esteem. The social interactions of exercise, doing things with someone else, in a group, or meeting afterwards, cannot be overstated. Exercise then can be part of life, enhancing it, not merely an 'add-on' to life.

Exercise helps with strength and stamina. There are plenty of ways to stay strong and fit, and we can select what works for *us*, to improve our 'engine' and condition our muscles for strength, suppleness and balance. This is important as we age – indeed exercise may benefit us *more* as we age. We don't get bodybuilder looks in our seventies and eighties, but our limbs work better, we are less frail and less likely to fall and break something, which is one of the preventable hazards of ageing. You really are never too old to get fit!

Exercise is a great way to improve insulin resistance. This is especially the case in muscles, which is good for getting blood glucose down and improving T2D. Remember too that insulin resistance plays a part in high blood pressure, artery disease and NAFLD, and they can all be helped by being more active. Secondly, exercise can boost and increase the number of the tiny energy generators in our cells – the mitochondria – which give us our sense of energy and make us feel more alive!

There is some evidence that lowering insulin resistance can improve the health of nerve cells, sharpen up our thinking and even slow down ageing in the brain. While all these good things are going on in the background, exercise also often improves our sleep, and we know how much better *that* makes us feel.

People say, 'I feel so much better when I am active' – and we can see why – another reminder of how everything about us is joined up!

You are several times more likely to develop T2D if you have a parent, brother, sister or child with the condition; even nephews and nieces are a little more likely to develop it. The genes which give us insulin-resistant muscles – a big part of that increased risk – can't be swapped, but we can blunt their effect by becoming and staying physically fit. Even if a close relative has T2D, we ourselves are protected by achieving and maintaining a healthy body weight and minimising the excess liver fat which can trigger the disease.

Pause for thought

How many of *your* relatives have T2D?

All the benefits of changing what we do to manage T2D, whether it's our way of eating or just being active, need to continue long-term to keep the benefit. If for some reason we had to stop, or we fell ill for example, we wouldn't lose the gains overnight, especially fitness which has some memory. But whether we are trying to be more active, exercise more or change our diet for the better, in order to work it will need to be sustained, which means making it an *enjoyable* part of our life. The health and fitness benefits of exercise stay with us – as long as we stay with it!

Exercise and weight loss

We've seen that exercise and being more active have the potential to make us all much healthier, but what about weight loss? Losing weight doesn't guarantee any health gain, just as being overweight doesn't necessarily make a person unhealthy. However, in T2D, weight loss and health are often intertwined and if you have T2D you almost certainly have to lose weight to make a big difference, like reversing the disease.

Is exercise a good way to lose weight? Disappointingly, it seems not. When scientists study people exercising to lose weight, there are some consistent observations:

- Some weight loss occurs and then tends to be regained, just as in dieting, and a similar on/off or yo-yo pattern can emerge.

- Without real determination and discipline, people tend to eat more when exercising – it's natural, and largely appetite-driven, but some conscious self-rewarding occurs.

- Exercise can be hard work for many of us, especially when starting up, and if weight loss is an aim, and little occurs, it can be demoralising. In some ways, exercise and dieting for weight loss can follow similar paths – enthusiasm declines.

Here is someone, however, whose enthusiasm for exercise did not decline.

Alan, 42, policeman

Alan saw his doctor after a routine work medical had picked up raised blood pressure and a slightly abnormal liver blood test. The medical report also carried a comment about his weight. A police inspector with no prior major health problems, Alan was fond of a night out with friends or work colleagues, but enjoyed jogging and the odd game of squash, which he felt balanced things out and helped with the stress of his job. His BMI was 29 – significantly overweight – and he was 10kg (22lb) heavier than in his mid-twenties, at the time he got married.

He drank alcohol 'in moderation', but his doctor pointed out that the actual amount was well above health guidelines!

Alan was happy with the plan to do some home monitoring of blood pressure and repeat his blood test including a screen for T2D. A month later, Alan's liver test was still slightly out of the normal range, and his diabetes screening test showed him to be at risk of T2D. Alan was surprised by his result but felt he had plenty of scope to make helpful changes. He thought the doctor's advice to turn the clock back fifteen years on his weight was a little excessive, and declined referral to a dietician, saying he would do a bit more exercise and cut down on his food portions.

Alan loved to run, it made him feel good, and he was convinced that it would be helping him burn off the calories from the food that he so loved. He had once joked to a friend, 'I run so that I can eat chips.' He wasn't quite sure why he continued to steadily put on weight in spite of running a good few miles a week. It was irritating to him.

Alan's experience is a conundrum shared by many. We don't associate regular exercise with weight gain. What can we make of it? What would you make of it?

Perhaps he was just taking in more calories than he was using. Perhaps he was eating the 'wrong' type of food or drinking too much alcohol. Perhaps exercise was making him eat more, and his belief that the more exercise he did, the more his weight *should* drop, was a kind of trap. Alan himself believed that without running his weight would have been even higher, or he might already have had T2D. Perhaps he needed to do even more?

There could be some truth in all of these reflections. The only certainties here were that three to four hours a week of moderate-to-strenuous exercise was not keeping his weight in check but that running made him feel good!

Alan had developed NAFLD and his liver had become insulin-resistant. Losing weight would be difficult without a dietary change. Exercise can bring some wonderful health benefits, but the one that we should least rely on is help with managing weight.

Exercise does make us *feel* much better, and it will help in T2D, but it's less likely to help with weight loss. Managing that expectation can help us stay with the health benefits that are more assured.

It took Alan a little while to get out of his trap, but once he had thought the problem through, he came round to accepting that he might have been wrong. It *wasn't* working. The impact of his diet on his weight, liver fat and glucose metabolism was overwhelming the good that exercise was otherwise doing for him. He didn't need to stop running, he just needed to find a way to lose weight that worked!

On the same theme, here is an observational experiment. If you watch an organised public run, such as one of the many half or full marathons that we can see in most cities and big towns around the world, you will see that the athletes at the front of the field are nearly all lean – slim or very slim. Then look at the remainder and you will see folk who are not much different in shape and size to those watching. You might think that the more athletic runners are used to running many more miles, which might be the main reason for their being slim.

However, top runners do not become lean by running longer distances – they were always slim. They run big miles *because* they are lean and have bodies which release energy easily (amongst other physical advantages), which makes running easier for them. Leanness facilitates exercise, not the other way round, which is the one disappointing myth around exercise. Think about this the next time you see people jogging in the streets or your local park.

Park and public runs are becoming popular these days, and what fantastic things they are, combining activity, fresh air and camaraderie. Jogging might not make us all slim but it can make everyone fitter, healthier, happier and probably live longer!

Children, and another lesson on exercise and weight

Researchers in the UK have found that weight gain in children occurred before they became less active, not, as we might think, the other way around. By following children over a long time period, scientists documented that children ate more first, then gained weight, then became less active – they were less inclined to play. This, of course, is exactly the opposite of the usual message put out by authorities and in government guidance, suggesting that getting children to exercise more is unlikely to help solve the childhood obesity crisis.

Children, like joggers, need to eat in a way that prevents weight gain, which also allows for easier energy release and more pleasurable exercise. Insulin resistance in children is the most worrying part of the pandemics of disease that we face. The future of T2D everywhere depends on children staying (mainly) lean and healthy.

So *why* might exercise not help us to lose weight? We think there are three compelling reasons:

Firstly, it's hard to do enough exercise to counter overeating; it can take an hour to burn the energy that it takes less than five minutes to eat. The effort in balancing calories doesn't work long-term.

Secondly, we talked about how the body will try to stop an attempt to change things – and it particularly values stored energy. It's a precious commodity and the body will try to hang on to it, frustrating though that may feel!

And finally, we get demoralised – it's hard work doing exercise, especially if our main aim is weight loss, and if it's not working then giving up is easy. We can reposition our take on this but then we have to get our head around being happy to be fit *without* losing weight.

Alan eventually changed his beliefs, which really helped him long-term.

We 'compensate' for the energy we burn during exercise

Important recent research shows that most of the energy we burn during exercise is compensated for by a reduction in background (autopilot) energy use. In other words, we don't turn all the burned calories from exercise into weight loss – in fact, possibly only 30–50 per cent (at most) depending on your size. Sadly, it turns out that the heavier we are, the more we compensate for the extra exercise and the harder it becomes to lose weight.

Both exercise and calorie reduction (conventional dieting) cause the body to adjust its internal controls to reduce background energy use. On top of that, the brain can coordinate hunger and food choices to subtly increase energy intake to compensate for what we use during exercise. The brain is effectively lowering the idling speed on our 'engine' and causing us to take a bit more fuel in to offset our weight loss attempts – it so wants us to hang on to stored energy (fat).

Neither exercise nor calorie reduction is useless for weight loss – they're just hard work. Research shows that exercise is better at helping maintain weight loss which has been achieved first by dietary means. Following the science means putting the emphasis on food changes first, then exercise. It's easier and works better!

For bedtime reading, here are some snippets from UK government guidance on how much exercise we need for health!

We can see from Figure 3.1 that the more we put in, the more benefit we can get. However, the slope of the line tells us that the 'return' is greatest at lower durations of exercise, so doing anything at all is hugely better than nothing!

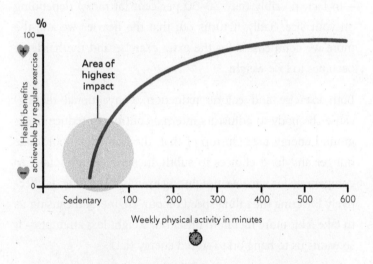

Figure 3.1: Health benefits connect with how much exercise we do

From UK Chief Medical Officers' guidance on exercise duration (2019). Guidance is similar around the world, and health benefits here include those most relevant to T2D.

For a modest ninety minutes a week we can get up to half of the available health gains. Standard guidance to do up to 150 minutes a week, or little more than twenty minutes a day, is aimed at giving us all about 75 per cent of the benefits for a modest outlay of time and effort.

Getting to near maximum benefit would take us about ten hours a week, so that last 25 per cent of gain would be at the expense of more than seven hours of time! Of course, if it's all pleasure and fits well in your life – why not!?

The health gains referred to are spread across the areas shown in the table below.

Figure 3.2: Moderate or strong evidence for health benefit

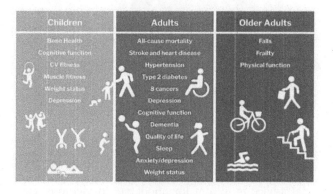

Children	Adults	Older Adults
Bone Health	All-cause mortality	Falls
Cognitive function	Stroke and heart disease	Frailty
CV fitness	Hypertension	Physical function
Muscle fitness	Type 2 diabetes	
Weight status	8 cancers	
Depression	Depression	
	Cognitive function	
	Dementia	
	Quality of life	
	Sleep	
	Anxiety/depression	
	Weight status	

The list of known benefits of exercise, from the UK Chief Medical Officers' Guidance published in 2019.

Some of the benefits come with a better diet, so a combination might be even more helpful. Figure 3.2 emphasises the wide benefits of exercise – from physical and mental health problems to physical and mental functioning, strength and resilience. Mood, tension, mental sharpness and sleep are all improved by exercising and being active.

Figure 3.3: How hard should we exercise?

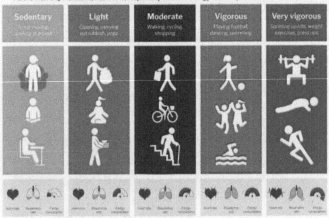

Intensity of exercise

As the intensity increases, heart rate, respiratory rate and energy consumption also increase further

*The benefits of different intensities of exercise,
from the UK Chief Medical Officers' Guidance
published in 2019.*

Official advice is to aim for 'moderate to vigorous' exercise, but almost anything can be made so by adjusting the speed or effort of what you do! Walking could be light, moderate or vigorous depending on the effort factor. A gentle cycle could be light to moderate, but preparation for the Tour de France would be vigorous to extreme. The basic rule of thumb is to be a little out of breath but able to speak and work up some sweat.

Pause for thought

Looking at Figure 3.3, how active are you? What kind of exercise, if any, do you engage in during an average week? How might you increase your activity each day? Make a list of realistic ways of doing this. How might you put this into action? Could you enlist the help of a friend or a family member to support you?

Does the type of exercise matter?

Probably not, but remember that exercise brings its benefits only when it's done regularly and long-term. So enjoyment is a big factor in choosing what to do. People say that the two most important things about any activity are to enjoy doing it and to ideally do it with someone else – which puts dancing and sex at the top of many people's lists!

If you really don't like to exercise or don't have someone to do it with, think about joining a gym group or class appropriate for your level or age. Use it as an opportunity to meet folk. Walking groups are an obvious and popular option. Doing something with other people is more enjoyable and may make you feel a little more committed too.

Benefits from exercise are not all to do with its physicality – feeling better can come from being confident, engaging with other people, and just having more human contacts and friendships.

If exercise hurts, use common sense – you may be doing the wrong thing for your body. For a lifelong runner, continuing into old age is probably OK, but taking it up at an age when the natural cushioning of cartilage in knees and hips is being lost might not be advisable. Not a problem with swimming, however; the water buoyancy helps muscles work without fuss, stretching and supporting joints. Ageing can be rolled back! We are all different and we each must find what works for us.

We are just starting to learn that combining different types of exercise can be helpful for health, weight and maybe for T2D. Mixing common aerobic activities – 'cardio' exercises, like walking, running, rowing, cycling or swimming – with muscle tensioning and strengthening exercises – typically push-ups, weights or machine-type activities – might increase fitness more than just doing one or another type alone. Gyms help the latter, but we can do much of this at home too with a mat and simple hand weights.

You may have heard of HIIT (high-intensity interval training), which is starting to gain attention in the diabetes world. It basically means doing an activity for a set time with varying levels of intensity within that time. It's simpler than it sounds and there is no rigid formula for it.

Let's use the example of an exercise bike, which is safe and can be accessed at home or in a gym. HIIT is founded on the principle that doing a series of short sprints (fast or hard pedalling to mimic going up a short hill) with longer recovery sections means you can get fitter more quickly than by just pedalling. The hard bits might last fifteen to thirty seconds, or longer if you are fitter. The recovery times are longer. There is obvious scope to build this up over a few weeks.

Individuals have reported some impressive results doing HIIT – including anecdotally reversing T2D – and the science makes sense. Varying the activity intensity can engage different muscles during the different intensities, and improves stamina and strength better than exercise sustained at the same level. It's also time-efficient – twenty minutes of HIIT might give the same benefit as an hour of regular exercise.

From a T2D point of view, HIIT may be especially advantageous:

- It appears to improve insulin resistance in our muscles, allowing for better use of glucose, which is good.

- The intense phases of exercise use a lot more glucose and help to run down glycogen – stored glucose – encouraging the body to burn more fat.

- It may be even more helpful to people who are overweight.

Using gym bikes, John cycles for 45 minutes at a steady pace. Pam joins him on the next machine and does 25 minutes of HIIT. By the time they finish Pam has used up significantly more energy than John and might have sharpened up her all-round fitness more. She is not more tired than John, but she is much more smug!

Scientific research on this form of exercise is still emerging, but we have enough knowledge to recommend that people think about this approach for T2D – it is promising.

Don't expect miracles, ideally research it first and get help from a trainer. Don't overdo it – it might be counterproductive and risking injury is to be avoided. Time will tell whether this really makes a major difference to T2D, so let's wait and see.

If you are new to exercise, don't worry about the latest fashions. To begin with, stick to basic principles – do what you enjoy, do things with others if possible, and do it from January to December!

What if I can't exercise?

Experts have found the benefits of exercise to be the same whether you have restrictions or are fully able-bodied. The same guidance applies and remember that, if you enjoy it, then the more you can do the better, but half an hour a day will do nicely. Apply common sense and exercise safely if you have problems with your hearing or vision.

Explore your options with family, friends or your doctor/nurse but, at the end of the day, exercise may not be for you or you might have such a severe restriction that you can barely move. If you lose weight, that's great, but don't worry if you can't. This is all about improving your general health, which can happen without weight loss.

Can exercise cause me any harm if I have T2D?

Essentially, no. You need to take care if you have physical restrictions or complications affecting your feet. If you are on medication that could make you prone to hypoglycaemia – especially insulin – you need to plan and prepare. But exercise will rarely cause harm if you are thoughtful. The benefits of exercise and being active will *always* outweigh, by far, any small challenges.

Bear in mind that Sir Steve Redgrave won five Olympic gold medals in rowing whilst on insulin!

When thinking about health and T2D, the way we eat, how active we are and how well we sleep all matter, and they all interlink. Sleeping well improves our eating patterns and how energetic we feel. Being more active helps us to sleep well and eating better can help us to stay active. We are all joined up! For T2D, regular exercise reduces:

- Insulin resistance.

- Liver fat.

- Blood pressure.

- The risk of artery disease.

- HbA1c.

And helps with:

- Psychological wellbeing.

- Better sleep.

- Maintaining a healthier weight.

- Maintaining reversal of T2D.

If you are planning a new T2D 'makeover' and want to improve your fitness and make a dietary change, then definitely change your eating first. Attempting to reverse T2D is a very big effort, and it's better to wait until you are properly adjusted (at least two or three months) before attempting more exercise. Ordinary steady walking is fine. Switching to a low-carbohydrate diet predictably needs two to four weeks to allow the 'fuel change' to take place in the body and for energy to return, so it is counter productive trying to exercise during that adjustment period. But by then you should feel more than ready!

Now that you've had a good chance to think about how active you are, and maybe about how active you would like to be, it's time to share some final reflections on what we think helps in the challenge of becoming more active.

Figure 3.4: Being more active

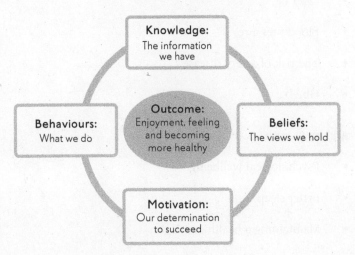

What things might help you to be more active and what things, if any, might be making you feel stuck? These are probably just opposite sides of the same coin.

Pause for thought

Take some time to think about the following questions:

- What do I know about exercise – do I need to ask or find out more?

- What do I think about exercise – will it really help?

- Am I up for it – am I going to give it my best shot?

- Is my body ready? For most people dietary weight loss first is a great help.

Once you have decided you want to be more active and be fitter – then go for it! You will know when exercising is helping because you will feel better, both mentally and physically. If you can feel *that*, the benefits are assured. When you have read about self-monitoring (Chapter 8), you might want to use a diary, over a few weeks or months, to track other aspects of how you are feeling such as your mood and sleeping – and how aspects of your T2D are shaping up. Blood pressure often falls with regular exercise and self-monitoring can give positive feedback, even within the first month.

Helping each other

We can't tell for sure how many of us are active enough. Surveys show tremendous variation around the world and over time. It's possible that the number of us who are insufficiently active might be as low as 25 per cent or as high as 80 per cent. Whatever the reality is, we can be sure that a lot of people are not getting the health benefits that they might, and a lot of us exercise in spells rather than regularly or long-term. Significant numbers of people never exercise.

Even when a person has not been able to maintain their weight, taking *plentiful* exercise can probably lower the major risks to health by as much as 50 per cent. It's hugely worthwhile and with few or no financial costs. No drug could give this level of benefit.

And yet, *not* exercising is, from an evolutionary perspective, the normal way to be. And if you stop and reflect on what we are all doing when we're exercising, it can seem genuinely strange if not downright weird. A time traveller looking at twenty-first-century human life would wonder what was going on!

- If you exercise regularly, carry on. You understand what this is all about. If you do it alone, encourage someone you know to join you.

- If you don't exercise, or could do more, think about those risk-free health gains.

- Remember that exercise can be difficult to start up, a drive to do it is not built into any of us.

- If you cannot get going, don't blame or shame yourself – you are normal; it might yet come to you.

Doing things with others, such as park runs, can be more enjoyable. We are more likely to keep it up and it can become second nature. The accruing benefits are hidden from view – the upfront ones are feeling brighter and better in ourselves, and having the energy to enjoy the rest of our lives.

Let's end this chapter on an exercise high! Margaret, who we met in Chapter 1, had a good introduction to exercise by her friend Neera. Margaret had never really been an exerciser; her work as a carer kept her on the move but her caseload was not very physically demanding.

Being diagnosed with T2D started to change her life. She had gained a lot of weight over many years and the nurse had, in a kindly way, suggested she had a choice: carry on as she was, and just medicate downwards her HbA1c if need be; or really give it a good go, meaning she'd have to work hard on her diet and fitness. After a few weeks, and losing a few pounds, she was taken to a gym class by Neera, which was a key point in her journey.

She struggled with some of the exercises and keeping up, but had a laugh, and met a couple of people she hadn't seen for years. The stiffness from the first classes soon wore off, and she looked forward to them more than she could have imagined. She started to play badminton with Neera and her other new friends, and a new social life blossomed from her diagnosis of T2D! Three months into her new regime, her HbA1c was almost down to fifty, (below forty-eight is non-diabetic). Of course, this was not all down to exercise. She was on one diabetes tablet a day and remained motivated to control her diet. Things were moving in the right direction again.

Key points from Chapter 3

- Although we evolved to be active, exercise is equally good for us.

- Being active makes us feel good; we have more energy and may sleep better.

- Being active can improve our mental health.

- Being more active can help prevent T2D.

- Exercise is not, on its own at least, a good way to lose weight but is better at helping to prevent weight regain.

- Exercise, like eating well, is for the long haul, so do what you enjoy, ideally with others.

Sleeping well to help T2D

FAST – introducing sleep

> *'If sleep and dreaming do not perform some vital biological function, then they must represent nature's most stupid blunder and most colossal waste of time.'*

Stevens (1997)

You would not be surprised to find a discussion about eating and exercise in a book about T2D. The links between T2D, weight and being fit and active are well embedded in us all, but where does sleep come in? How does it affect physical and mental health, and how does that fit with T2D?

All living beings sleep or have sleep-like mechanisms, which alone tells us that sleep is rooted in the evolution of life and must therefore have a key role in its processes. Because sleep is 'of' the brain (in humans at least), the organ that controls and coordinates metabolism, it should not surprise us that we are finding links between sleep and life's basic functions – including with metabolism itself. We now know too that life simply does not work without sleep; it is a necessity, like air, fuel and water. Without it we die.

The nature of sleep – we are offline but not switched off!

How many of us have stopped to think why we spend up to a third of our lives unconscious, with not the slightest clue as to what we are actually doing in that twilight world of sleep? If we pause to reflect, we probably imagine that somehow both body and mind simply need to refresh and reset.

For most of us, sleep is a positive thing – we enjoy the feeling of approaching sleep, as we tire and get ready for bed. It's good to know we are entering a relaxed place, and can look forward to feeling rested and refreshed. The mind can be closed down, with thoughts dispelled or tucked away. But while the mind is resting, the brain itself is far from shut down, and it may be even busier in some ways than it is when we are awake! We don't just sleep to rest from thinking. So why do we sleep? Perhaps the question should be, 'Why does all life need the things that sleep brings?' And also, 'Why is sleep so strongly linked to light and dark – to the essential rhythm of life on our planet?' Thankfully, we don't have to fully answer those big questions here! But they are becoming increasingly relevant to understanding diseases of the way the body works, like T2D, and we'll touch on why that matters in this chapter.

Metabolism and maintenance. Sleep does so much more than rest metabolism and save a little energy. Many of the crucial background processes that keep us healthy happen when we are asleep. The body's repair and maintenance systems can move into action when the body is quiet and less occupied with managing energy balance. We make a lot of important chemicals overnight when the body is also busy repairing itself. The immune system – the fighter of illness and infection – is weighted towards the sleep hours. 'You'll feel better after a good night's sleep' is not just a saying.

From a T2D perspective, it is helpful to bear in mind that the internal chemical controls of metabolism – which include insulin – are not just linked to sleep itself but to the daily clock systems within the brain which govern the release of these substances. So for health, sleep is important in itself, but so is the timing of the sleep in relation to the body's natural time settings.

Help with thinking and memory. That part of nightly maintenance that moves into action in the brain overnight helps to clear nerve tissue of a build-up in materials which can form tangles and inflammation around the brain cells themselves. In the parts of the brain concerned with storing knowledge, sleep helps us to consolidate new information – things that we have taken on board during the previous day. It oversees the ordered internal filing of new items to help us with recall – in other words, our memory.

The brain regulates metabolism, just as it regulates everything else, and we now know that a lot of that regulating is going on while we are asleep and at night. When we are sleeping well we don't pay attention to it. Why would we? But we certainly take notice when we sleep badly.

When sleep is impaired. We have always been aware of a link between mental health problems and poor sleep. We struggle to get to sleep when feeling anxious – rumination and a busy head are not helpful. When we are depressed, we can struggle with all phases of sleep, with waking early a common pattern. But we are now becoming aware of the potential for poor sleep to bring on, or worsen, physical health problems, especially those involving metabolic health. Sleep problems are as strongly linked with T2D as they are with depression, and the whole range of related problems we've been discussing seem to be impacted by short or poor-quality sleep.

Pause for thought

Think for a moment on when you last missed a night's (or a big part of a night's) sleep. Think how you felt the following day, and what you did to manage that.

Most of the time, we don't worry when things like that happen because we know that things get back to normal quickly. However, scientists who have studied those short periods of sleep loss tell us that they affect us much more than we think. Judgement and decision-making are substantially impaired. Have you ever stopped to think whether you should be behind the wheel of a car after a poor night's sleep? No? Studies show that missing sleep impairs the brain as much, if not more than, drinking alcohol. While most of us would think twice about driving with a hangover, we might not if we felt tired from a lack of sleep, which is just as hazardous!

We said good sleep supports memory and the opposite, inadequate sleep, definitely impairs it. For example, a study of healthy students in 2006 found a 50 per cent decreased recall of paired lists of words with one night of four hours of sleep compared to eight hours. We don't know for sure if poor sleep contributes long-term to dementia, but some scientists think it may be a factor.

Normal or healthy sleep. When we think of a good night's sleep, we aspire to getting eight hours, but is this a myth? Seven to eight hours is simply an average for connection with good health, but there is a large variation in normal amounts of sleep needed at different ages.

Figure 4.1, redrawn from a National Sleep Foundation study, shows a large variation in normal amounts of sleep needed at any age. Healthy sleep duration for young adults might be around seven to nine hours, and seven to eight hours for older people – bear in mind, as the table shows, it's possible to be healthy outside these ranges. You have a healthy sleep schedule if you sleep consistently, feel rested and refreshed, and are free of physical and mental health problems.

The amount we sleep changes over our life. We could go from needing ten hours of sleep at twenty to less than six hours over the age of sixty-five. Sometimes when we get older, we chase sleep that we don't actually need. Although John would say he has always been an early riser, Pam was a confirmed night owl for most of her life but has noticed a change in recent years to becoming a lark. One of the perks of getting older – we are awake longer and we all become larks!

Figure 4.1: How much sleep do we need?

National Sleep Foundation
Recommended Sleep Durations

Age	Hours of Sleep																			
	1	2	3	4	5	6	7	8	9	10	11	12	13	14	15	16	17	18	19	20
Older Adult ≥65 years	1	2	3	4	5	6	7	8	9	10	11	12	13	14	15	16	17	18	19	20
Adult 26–64 years	1	2	3	4	5	6	7	8	9	10	11	12	13	14	15	16	17	18	19	20
Young Adult 18–25 years	1	2	3	4	5	6	7	8	9	10	11	12	13	14	15	16	17	18	19	20
Teenager 14–17 years	1	2	3	4	5	6	7	8	9	10	11	12	13	14	15	16	17	18	19	20
School age 6–13 years	1	2	3	4	5	6	7	8	9	10	11	12	13	14	15	16	17	18	19	20

	1	2	3	4	5	6	7	8	9	10	11	12	13	14	15	16	17	18	19	20
Preschool 3–5 years	1	2	3	4	5	6	7	8	9	10	11	12	13	14	15	16	17	18	19	20
Toddler 1–2 years	1	2	3	4	5	6	7	8	9	10	11	12	13	14	15	16	17	18	19	20
Infant 4–11 months	1	2	3	4	5	6	7	8	9	10	11	12	13	14	15	16	17	18	19	20
Newborn 0–3 months	1	2	3	4	5	6	7	8	9	10	11	12	13	14	15	16	17	18	19	20

Recommended Range

May be appropriate

Not Recommended

What is poor sleep? What do we *mean* by poor sleep – less total sleep or poorer, more disturbed sleep? Both the duration and quality of sleep can impact our health, with some studies suggesting that the latter may even be worse for us. Sleeping only four or five hours or less a day may mean you have a connected health problem. But sleeping longer than nine, certainly ten hours, might also be a sign of a health problem, and can also be linked with taking particularly sedative types of medication.

The message is becoming more and more clear – sleep is not a minor player in staying well. It is not just an option to choose if we have the time to fit it in; a luxury as it were. It is an essential part of the way we all stay healthy. We don't know how all things physical and mental connect with sleep, just that they do.

We have long realised that physical and mental health problems intertwine. Now we know that both are linked with sleep problems which might well play a big role in that intertwining.

Sleep, sleep deprivation and T2D. We have known for some time that sleep deprivation is associated with an increased risk of T2D and other related conditions, like high blood pressure and artery disease. Furthermore, small but controlled experiments in sleep laboratories have confirmed that insufficient or poor-quality sleep most definitely has adverse effects on insulin and glucose metabolism. One study showed that such changes – up to the level of someone at risk of T2D – could be brought about in healthy people by limiting sleep to four or five hours per day *for just a week!* And you are significantly more likely to develop T2D itself if you are deprived of sleep long-term.

So we know then that poor or short sleep, along with other lifestyle issues, can contribute to a person's risk of getting T2D. But how?

Firstly, by increasing insulin resistance. Poor sleep impedes the way we manage glucose, via the neural (nerve) connections from the brain to the liver. Sleep and brain function are intimately connected; the brain manages insulin overall, so if sleep is the body's way of tuning and resetting things on a daily basis, we might not be surprised that a lack of it might impact on the body's chemistry.

Secondly, by increasing the sensation of hunger through complex hormonal and chemical messengers. Poor sleep makes us eat more but feel less satisfied, and a lack of energy makes us less active. The signalling of hunger is significantly impaired when we are sleep deprived. The extra food we eat tends to be carbohydrates – particularly sugar – and much more so than fat- or protein-rich foods. Scientists have seen MRI scan changes which might lie behind these food choices; parts of the brain where conscious thinking and judgement are formed are seen to be less active when we lack good sleep, while deeper areas of the brain concerned with gratification or reward are more active. It seems that when we sleep badly, we choose biscuits over nuts every time!

Why do we sleep only or mainly at night?

The circadian rhythm – from the Latin *circa* and *diem* (literally 'around a day') – is the name for the natural, timed processes that occur each day in living things. Preparation for being active, to take in food, and to rest and sleep are all based on a light-sensitive part of the brain, and a very long period of evolution!

Mammals generally sleep in consistent spells during the light/dark cycle of each day. Some mammals are nocturnal and are evolved to be active at night-time. Humans, like dogs, are diurnal creatures, and are programmed to be active in daylight. We sleep naturally at night because our brain's 'clock', which governs the behaviour of our chemistry, and therefore our systems and activities, sets the sleep/wake rhythm of our body in the diurnal pattern. It seems that to get the best from sleep's health-promoting effects, including a healthy metabolism, we need to sleep in tune with nature.

Science has demonstrated that sleeping sufficiently for health – call it seven to eight hours – matters, but it seems to be equally important that we sleep *when we are meant to sleep*. Short-term upsets to our sleep/wake cycle, such as jet lag from a long-haul flight, are a nuisance, but we generally slip back into our usual sleep pattern without much difficulty after a couple of days. This is not the case with ongoing rotational shift work when sleep patterns change frequently. This is when health problems can arise.

Mustafa, 54, factory worker

Mustafa worked in a car factory which operated a shift system of work. He had an annual medical review of his blood pressure, which had been a problem for a few years. In his late forties, Mustafa had started to work shifts, following a change in company policy. The factory operated three shifts: early from 6 a.m. to 2 p.m., late from 2 p.m. to 10 p.m., and night from 10 p.m. to 6 a.m. Rotation through the shift phases, every few weeks, was expected.

At the age of fifty-one, his blood pressure medication had been increased, and his weight started to rise. His blood glucose was slightly higher and his HbA1c reached 45mmol/mol – putting him significantly at risk of T2D, especially with his rising weight.

Night shift working makes it hard to get enough quality sleep. The world in the daytime is lighter, noisier and busier. Things are happening that we may want to be part of and we are hardwired to be awake during the day and asleep at night.

The detrimental impacts of poor sleep are then compounded by sleeping at the 'wrong time' of the day, which scientists have found doubles the harmful impact on metabolism for shift workers. Moreover, these impacts seem to be made even worse by frequently *changing* shift times.

We can be certain that the risk of gaining weight and of developing T2D is significantly increased by shift work and its adverse effects on metabolism; if night shift working cannot be avoided, *regularising* rather than rotating shifts lessens the risk.

We will come back to Mustafa in Chapter 8 when we look at another challenging variation on usual day/night functioning – that of religious fasting (Ramadan), which became a more complex issue for Mustafa when he developed T2D and later started insulin treatment.

Thinking about your own sleep

If you have a bad night's sleep, or even two, it will affect you, but you don't necessarily need to change your routines – just understand it, work it out and tolerate it. If you feel you need to catch up from a sleepless night, you don't need to sleep for double the length of time the next night, it's about a third extra (one-and-a-third night's worth) that is needed to catch up.

If it's an obvious source of worry, talk it through with someone close to you if you can. If sleep has been a problem for a while, or the cause is ongoing, then try some (or ideally all) of the tips later in this chapter.

Complete a sleep diary

Like all diaries, you can make your own or use one of the many available online. The sleep diary in Appendix 3: Resources (for Chapter 4) is from *How to Beat Insomnia and Sleep Problems* (Anderson, 2023) with permission of Little, Brown Book Group. Complete the diary each day for at least ten days, ideally two weeks. Keep it nearby (with a pen) and record entries, preferably each morning (not at night).

Like all self-monitoring (Chapter 8), a diary provides you with real-time information, rather than estimation (guesswork), and allows you to assess your overall sleep duration and quality. You might even find that you don't sleep as badly as you think. We all sometimes think we've hardly slept at all, but we have. Include extra information in the diary such as: alcohol, caffeinated drinks (for example coffee, tea, hot chocolate, cola), any sleep medication, meals, snacks, exercise, going to the toilet, noise that disturbs you, time of wake-up alarm (if you use one), sleep time (including naps), and any glucose readings if you self-monitor. Keeping a diary like this will allow you to spot any obvious associations between sleep and other possible connected factors. And, like all self-monitoring, if you tackle it purposefully and thoroughly it is likely to help you improve your sleep.

You may be using your phone, watch or other gadget to monitor your sleep. But beware, apps and gadgets have been found to over-score movement as a sign of being awake, when the person is actually moving while asleep. In addition to their inaccuracy, because using apps or gadgets is a marker of being awake, it is recommended they are avoided. For the monitoring period you may find Dr Anderson's diary helps you capture the information more accurately. More on the pros and cons of sleep apps later.

Once you have completed monitoring for a couple of weeks, review the diaries. What can you learn about your sleep? Was your sleep affected by any known factors, such as light, noise, nicotine, caffeine, etc.? What did you learn from the exercise that you can change to help improve your sleep?

Check your diary for the following:

- Any daytime napping.

- Going to the loo to pee during the night.

- Caffeine and alcohol.

- Timing of any medication.

- Variability (occasional good nights).

- Patterns in blood glucose readings if done.

- Total sleep time compared to time spent in bed (sleep efficiency – see below).

If you go to bed at 11 p.m. and get up at 7 a.m., that is eight hours in bed. But if you only sleep for four of those hours, that is 50 per cent sleep efficiency. Using your sleep diaries, calculate your own sleep efficiency across a week by adding up the total amount of time you were asleep over seven nights and dividing by seven for your average total sleep time (TST). Then add up the time you spent in bed (TIB). You then divide the TST by the TIB and express as a percentage.

Suzanne had an average TST of five hours (300 minutes). Her average time in bed was 8.5 hours (510 minutes). So Suzanne's sleep efficiency was 300 divided by 510 = 0.59 or 59 per cent. What does that tell us about Suzanne's sleep? Most adults will have a sleep efficiency of 85–90 per cent, which means that Suzanne's is some way off. We'll look at how to improve sleep efficiency a little later.

Pause for thought

How does your sleep efficiency compare with the adult average of 85–90 per cent? If it is below 85 per cent you may benefit from some of the strategies in this chapter.

We are always in one of three states of consciousness: awake; non-rapid eye movement (NREM) sleep; or rapid eye movement (REM) sleep. None of us sleeps through the night without waking – this is very important to be aware of. Everyone wakes up several times during the night. Most of us don't remember waking, but we all do it and it can be as many as ten to twelve times by the time we are over sixty. If you wake up and it feels like a long time (say fifteen minutes or so), that's insomnia. Here's what a night of sleep looks like:

Non-REM sleep. This happens first. There are three stages of non-REM sleep, with Stage 1 being the lightest. If you wake someone from Stage 1 sleep they often don't realise they were asleep. The sleep becomes deeper as we go through the stages, with Stage 3 of non-REM sleep being the deepest (sometimes referred to as slow wave sleep or delta sleep). During this stage, body temperature and heart rate fall and our brains use less energy. This is the stage of sleep that tends to create that feeling of being refreshed in the morning and having experienced a good night's sleep.

REM sleep. This takes a smaller portion of our total sleep time and is when we dream, which is associated with fast brain waves, eye movement and loss of muscle tone.

The full sleep cycle. A full cycle of sleep, moving through the stages of non-REM and REM sleep, takes around ninety minutes and we do this up to six times a night, sometimes more when we are older. Going through these stages of sleep up to six or more times means that there are variations in consciousness levels throughout the night. There will be periods of waking even in a good night's sleep, but the sleeper is unlikely to remember. Some people with disturbed sleep find that they wake around ninety minutes into their sleep. This marks the completion of the first sleep cycle as the person moves from non-REM and REM sleep, and is therefore normal.

Pause for thought

Does learning that this cycle is part of normal sleep and nothing to be concerned about in itself help to reduce anxiety about your sleep?

In a typical normal night's sleep, it takes about twenty to thirty minutes to fall into NREM sleep and you will feel groggy if woken up. We move in cycles through the stages of sleep, with the amount of REM sleep (when we will have vivid dreams) increasing in the two cycles just before natural awakening. See Figure 4.2 for a typical night's sleep. The grey blocks in the diagram show how dream sleep increases throughout the night. That's why, if an alarm clock wakes you up, you may remember a dream. (NB: N1–3 are the stages of non-REM sleep.)

Figure 4.2: Hypnogram of normal sleep

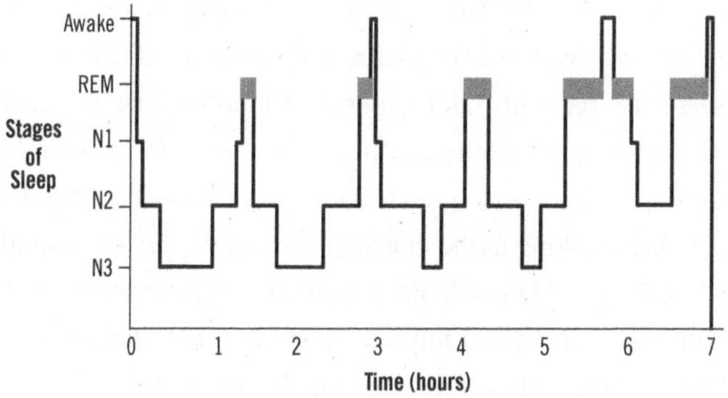

Reproduced from Anderson, How to Beat Insomnia and Sleep Problems *(2023), with permission from Little, Brown Book Group.*

Interestingly, we are most wakeful in the two hours before sleep, so it is no wonder that if we go to bed early to get more sleep, we find we are wide awake!

Physical health and sleep

Sleep has a complex relationship with illness and almost any long-term condition can impair sleep. Particularly troublesome are conditions that cause pain – for example musculoskeletal conditions including arthritis – and those causing breathlessness, such as heart failure or chronic obstructive pulmonary disease (COPD). Discuss the management of any condition that you feel may be affecting your sleep with your healthcare team/doctor, as there are often options that can help.

One very common and intrusive disturber of sleep is obstructive sleep apnoea (OSA). This condition is strongly linked to having T2D, obesity, high blood pressure and an increased risk of artery disease. People with OSA experience loud snoring associated with pauses in breathing causing wakening and a very broken night's sleep. The person can feel like they haven't had any sleep at all, often waking in the morning with a sore, dry throat and a dull headache. They will almost certainly experience excessive daytime sleepiness and impaired concentration, and are likely to find it difficult to get through the day without having a nap. Snoring by itself is not a sign of OSA, and not everyone with OSA snores, but when severe and persistent snoring is accompanied by the other features described here, OSA is highly likely, so one to definitely discuss with your doctor.

Recent research suggests that OSA may be more common than we thought, with between 10 and 30 per cent of all people affected (and not just adults). The number of people estimated to have OSA worldwide is around 1 billion – similar to the number affected by high blood pressure, obesity and NAFLD, and about twice the number of people with T2D. Rising rates of OSA are closely tracking metabolic disease so, as we might expect, it is increasing everywhere, especially in men. Recent research suggests that one in three American men might have OSA. It's thought that the majority of people with OSA are undiagnosed.

> **Pause for thought**
>
> If you have T2D, you are much more likely to have OSA (and vice versa). Might any of the features of OSA apply to you? If you sleep with someone else, have they raised any concerns?

It's estimated that as many as half of all people with T2D have sleep problems, including insomnia, due to unstable blood glucose levels and accompanying diabetes-related symptoms, especially getting up to go to the toilet more often. You might benefit from self-monitoring blood glucose (Chapter 8), and a discussion within your care team could help.

Sleep tips: simple adjustments that nearly everyone agrees can help

Key strategies for a good night's sleep include:

1. Only go to bed when sleepy – that might seem obvious, but many of us go to bed when we are bored or feeling

weary or tired. That is not the same as being sleepy. More on this a little later.

2. Try to ensure that your bedroom is cool, dark and quiet. Heating should be low/off in the bedroom. If there is street lighting outside the window then blackout blinds or an eye mask can help. Loud street noise can be reduced with ear plugs. Any clocks should not be visible to help avoid counting down to getting up, and sleep experts recommend keeping smartphones and tablets out of view, preferably out of the room. They are associated with wakeful activities and light, which can obstruct the brain's sleep settings. If you have a problem with sleep you might want to bear this in mind, or simply compare periods of sleep with and without your phone/app to see what works best for you. Staying out of the bedroom during the day strengthens the connection between bed and night-time sleep. Don't do anything else in the bedroom apart from sleep, dress/undress and have sex!

3. Avoid eating within an hour or two of bedtime – it increases the chances of waking soon after getting off to sleep. In addition, our night-time physiology is set for us to sleep, not to eat; evidence consistently suggests that late evening eating (especially of the main meal) drives weight gain, raising insulin resistance and blood glucose.

4. What we do in the last hour or so before bed can influence our ability to sleep. Working late, thinking about work or the things that need to be done the next day, can

add to a racing mind (more on a racing mind later in the chapter) or feeling awake. It's best to stop working at least one hour before bed.

5. A bedtime routine helps us prepare for sleep and is an opportunity to unwind from the stresses of the day. In the hour before bed, try doing something quiet and relaxing like reading, listening to a podcast or watching television. A predictable bedtime routine can help the onset of sleep and can include activities like brushing teeth, setting the alarm, applying creams, closing the curtains, etc. Good sleepers tend to have a set bedtime routine, so it is a good idea to establish one.

6. Take some exercise in the day – ideally early on – and combine that with getting outdoor sunlight for at least thirty minutes (this matters more than you think), so a morning walk is ideal. Any moderate (or more) exercise will help sleep overall but, again, avoid in the last one or two hours before bed.

7. Reduce or avoid caffeine and alcohol (see later).

8. If you smoke, reduce this if you can. It will improve your chances of sleeping better, lower your risk from T2D (Chapter 7) and the impacts of lung disease and OSA.

9. Be thoughtful about using napping as a strategy (see later).

10. If you are on regular medication, whether prescribed or bought over the counter, think about whether it might

affect sleep, read the leaflet (some medications include caffeine), or talk to the pharmacist – changing the time you take tablets can be a quick fix!

Napping. This is a little contentious, and both research and expert opinion suggest using common sense. Some believe that we might have evolved to sleep in two spells during each twenty-four-hour period – the main one being at night. But modern life makes it difficult for many of us to follow any hardwiring for an early afternoon nap. If you have problems sleeping at night, napping should be avoided, so work at finding a night-time solution first. But if you sleep well, short naps of up to thirty minutes by early afternoon are not likely to be detrimental and might even be healthy. Guidance really depends on whether you have a sleep problem (insomnia) or not. Research on napping is currently active, so watch this space.

Caffeine. Five or more cups of coffee a day, regardless of the time they are consumed, causes caffeine to reach a steady state in the bloodstream that can affect sleep. Cutting down on the number of cups of coffee a day is just as important as not drinking caffeinated drinks later in the evening. One can of regular cola equals an espresso. Note: decaffeinated coffee is not caffeine-free, rather it is lower in caffeine. Regular tea contains caffeine, as do a number of other drinks such as hot chocolate and numerous medications. If you are having sleep problems, it is a good idea to cut down your caffeine intake and to avoid it from early afternoon onwards. It can make a surprising difference.

Alcohol. Only natural sleep brings the health benefits we all want to see – 'medicating' sleep using alcohol does not, and can have major downsides.

Let's revisit Suzanne, whose mother had T2D. Suzanne had gained weight throughout her thirties and developed T2D in her forties after suffering from stress and depression. A difficult house move had led to her using alcohol to try to relieve her stress and poor sleep. However, she admitted later that her strategy had backfired – both problems actually worsened. She began to wake progressively earlier, and felt more and more tired, sometimes 'comfort-snacking' as she called it, during the night.

Alcohol causes problems for people with depression and T2D separately, and together even more so. Although we associate alcohol with falling asleep, it is sedative, not natural, sleep, so the usual benefits are missing. Lighter broken sleep with vivid dreams is common. It may trigger a pattern of earlier waking, either because we need to go to the toilet or the alcohol sedation is wearing off during the night (or both). As it goes through our system, alcohol has depressant effects, doing exactly the opposite of what a person really needs.

It also brings unneeded calories and increases liver fat. A worsening of insulin resistance causes extra hunger, often leading to poor food choices, especially sweet food (comfort) snacking. We lose some of our sense of energy and become less active. In the background, glucose may be rising. Persistent poor sleep 'medicated' with alcohol impairs metabolism both in the brain and the liver.

All these factors will have contributed to Suzanne's worsening health – and pushed her from being at risk of T2D to actually having it. Alcohol is an understandable go-to when we are struggling, but when it comes to disturbed sleep and T2D, it's best avoided altogether.

Regarding sleeping medication, in his novel *The Holy*, American author Daniel Quinn compared sleeping pills to lies: 'You should only use them when you absolutely have to. They spoil everything if you make a habit of them.' Seeing your doctor about poor sleep is an option, but expect to talk and not be given a prescription for sleeping medication. The doctor will usually offer self-help information to begin with or a psychological therapy referral rather than medication. Cognitive behavioural therapy (CBT) has proven to be better than sleep medication, which in any event nowadays tends to be prescribed only short-term following a distressing or traumatic event.

Next steps: strengthening the link between the bed and sleep – the triple S

Once you have been keeping a diary for a couple of weeks and you have put in place the sleep tips, you may have noticed an improvement in your sleep. The following three steps have also been shown to be helpful. You might want to give them a go.

1. Sleep scheduling. Whilst regularising sleeping habits – including when you go to bed – can help you to maintain healthy sleep, if you have insomnia the important thing to decide first is what time you want to get up in the morning. What would work best with your daily routine? Once you decide on a time, stick to it. You might find it useful to set an alarm. No lie-ins at the weekend. It is vital that you commit to this. This is a seven-day-a-week regime going forward. It sounds tough, but so is living with insomnia, and these strategies have been found by researchers to work well.

Consider the following question: do you feel sleepy when you go to bed? This might seem like an obvious question, but sometimes we go to bed for other reasons such as being bored or feeling weary, or because it feels like the rest of the world has gone to bed. It can feel lonely being up late at night. Maybe you feel sleepy on the sofa, but as soon as you go to bed and turn the light off, it feels like one has been switched on in your head! So although it may seem an obvious question, many people do not go to bed when they feel sleepy and end up agitated and frustrated once in bed. What you are asked to do is not to go to bed until you are very, very sleepy (almost like a nodding dog). It is very important not to fix a bedtime if you have insomnia.

2. Sleep restriction. Let's look at what it would be like to aim for 90 per cent sleep efficiency. That may be far from where you are at the moment, but it is attainable. No pain, no gain with this one though. If you did the exercise earlier with examining your sleep diaries, you will already know your sleep efficiency. If not, use your diaries to see how much time you are awake during the night compared to the time you spend in bed, and make a note of your sleep efficiency. Lying in bed wide awake and agitated or cross about it only makes things worse. The aim of sleep restriction is to decrease time in bed awake and increase sleepiness and sleep efficiency. Suzanne's sleep efficiency was 59 per cent and she was averaging five hours of sleep a night.

Firstly, you will already have fixed your get-up time. To reduce frustration about not getting to sleep, try going to bed later. Sometimes we think we need more sleep than we do, and remember that the older we get, the less sleep we might need. Rather than continue to go to bed at 11 p.m., Suzanne agreed to go to bed at 12.30 a.m. It felt brutal, and the thought of doing it was horrid, but the current situation wasn't great either and because it was only for a couple of weeks at most, Suzanne decided to give it a go. This is a tough task to agree to, and even tougher to see it through, so planning is needed. The thing to remember is that the aim is to reduce frustration and strengthen the link between bed and sleep. The idea is to use what you have learned from your monitoring diaries to see how much sleep you usually get and set your bedtime to that time, even if it is 1.30 a.m. If it turns out that you need to reset the time to earlier, then do that by fifteen minutes at a time, but the idea is to minimise the time you are lying awake and maximise your time sleeping. Remember, if insomnia is getting you down and making you miserable, then this approach, although tough, has been proven to work, so it is definitely worth a try. What is important is that you do not restrict your sleep to being shorter than five hours.

You are likely to need some encouragement and support during this time, so do tell someone close to you what you are doing, and get their support, whether that be a friend, family member or partner. Sleep restriction has been shown to be the most effective strategy for reducing periods of wakefulness during the night – commit to trying it for one week in the first instance. If it is helping, do it for another week.

3. Stimulus control. We know that, in insomnia, the bed can become a place where people lie awake feeling frustrated about the inability to relax and get off to sleep. This can lead to feelings of dread about going to bed, as the expectation is for another bad night's sleep. Stimulus control is about taking the agitation out of the bedroom. It is frustrating and lonely being awake at 3 a.m. To help with this, consider:

The fifteen-minute rule. If you do not fall asleep within about fifteen minutes, get up and go into another room if possible, such as a quiet, warm space – perhaps on the sofa with a blanket and dim lighting. But avoid clock-watching – there shouldn't be one in sight – instead, notice if you are starting to feel frustrated and agitated about being wide awake. Do something relaxing, like reading a book (you are more likely to feel like dropping off reading a book than reading on a gadget) or listening to a podcast, doing a puzzle or reading a magazine. Television is best avoided as programmes are generally in chunks of thirty minutes or longer. Only go back to bed when you feel sleepy. Although it can be a struggle to get up in the middle of the night, you are more likely to get back to sleep sooner than lying awake feeling anxious about it. Do not work, clear a cupboard, clean or do anything active during this time.

If, after a couple of weeks, you are finding that you are feeling tired and getting to sleep within a few minutes of getting into bed and then sleeping through the night, start extending your time in bed by getting into bed fifteen minutes earlier for a few nights. If you are still falling asleep quickly, bring it back by another fifteen minutes. Keep on monitoring using the sleep diary to check you are quickly falling asleep. Keep on doing that until you find it is taking you a little longer to get to sleep, to find your 'sleep window' as you discover exactly how much sleep you need each night. It means you've found your sweet spot. If this doesn't work, why might that be? It may be that you are missing some of the steps, or it may be that you have another reason why you aren't sleeping. If you continue to have sleep problems do speak to your doctor, who will be able to advise and possibly refer you to someone who can help.

Slowing down a racing mind

Once you have all the other strategies in place, now is a good time to look at what you do with a busy head. Do you find that you are looking back over the day and planning the next day? Are you thinking about not sleeping and what it will mean to have another bad night? A racing mind is really just part of being awake – it is happening in the wrong place and at the wrong time. Instead, try running another programme, and no, it doesn't involve counting sheep! Try one or all of these strategies until you find the one that helps most. The knack is for them to be emotionless and have some complexity (counting sheep is not complex enough).

Putting the day away. If you find yourself thinking about the day that has just been and all that you need to do the next day, 'putting the day away' can be a useful technique. Try setting aside fifteen minutes at least two or three hours before bedtime. This task takes place away from the bedroom, in a normal waking space like the living room or at the kitchen table. You use a notebook or electronic equivalent to make a short list of what has happened in the day and what you did, and anything that you hoped to do but did not manage to. Next, write a short to-do list for the next day in the order the tasks should be done. This is a list for the next day only, not for the week or month. The list should be short and manageable. Also, check your diary so no thoughts about a forgotten arrangement/meeting, etc., will pop into your mind in the middle of the night.

Once you have completed the list and feel content that it is under control, put it away. Later, as it gets towards bedtime, you can remind yourself that you have put the day away. This can help tackle some of the worries that might contribute to a racing mind during the night.

Might you benefit from putting the day away? If so, try it out for three nights. Make a note of anything you learn from putting your day away.

Sleep-inducing techniques

Here are some techniques to use in bed which can help induce sleep. They can take a little practice and some may appeal more than others. You can chop and change across techniques as you like. More detail on these techniques can be found in *How to Beat Insomnia and Sleep Problems*, referred to earlier. They include:

Visualisation. Think of a fruit and think about it in great detail. Once you have it very clearly in mind, slowly change the colour of the fruit. The idea is that as you go through the various colours, this will help you go to sleep.

Verbal techniques. Think through a word category such as countries, different types of animals, breeds of dogs, cities, etc. For instance, if you decide on animals, go with the first animal that pops into your mind, say a hedgehog. Then think of another animal that begins with the last letter of that animal, so gorilla, armadillo, orangutan, and so on. The idea is to keep working through the sequence of words. It doesn't matter at all if you get any wrong or get stuck and have to restart. It is simply a way of creating a stream of words that doesn't have any emotion attached. Many people find this activity induces sleep.

Number techniques. Start with the number 1,000 and take away seven over and over and keep on going down by seven. Again, it does not matter if you make a mistake – and take it from us, that is likely!

Any of these techniques can be useful for a racing mind, or if you start to feel agitated or bothered about not getting off to sleep. The aim is to ensure that you do not start getting agitated about not sleeping. Over the next three nights, try each one of the sleep-inducing techniques (one per night) when you are ready to fall asleep. Do you find one easier to do than others? Which is your favourite?

Progressive muscle relaxation

Some people experience muscle tension and tossing and turning in bed. Most forms of formal relaxation are based on variations of progressive muscle relaxation. Below is a typical relaxation routine based on a sequence of exercises taken directly, with permission, from *The CBT Handbook* (Myles & Shafran, 2016). It is best to practise this first outside the bedroom. Once you get the hang of it, you can use the relaxation technique in bed at night.

Instructions: This relaxation exercise involves tensing and then relaxing various muscle groups. Work your way through your body, tensing each of the muscle groups below and holding for ten seconds each time.

1. Lower arms: tighten your fists and pull them up towards your body.

2. Upper arms: tense your arms by the side of your body.

3. Lower legs: extend your legs and point your feet up.

4. Upper legs: push your legs together.

5. Stomach: pull your stomach in towards your spine.

6. Upper chest and back: inhale and hold for a count of ten seconds.

7. Shoulders: pull your shoulders up towards your ears.

8. Back of the neck: tilt your head back.

9. Lips: purse your lips but without clenching your teeth.

10. Eyes: tightly close your eyes.

11. Eyebrows: frown, and push your eyebrows together.

12. Upper forehead: raise your eyebrows.

Remember to release each part of the body after ten seconds. You can do this exercise while sitting or lying down. It is a good idea to practise this exercise a few times.

If you have put into practice every aspect of the instructions in this chapter, you will have worked extremely hard over the last few weeks and will hopefully be reaping some rewards with improved sleep. Let's now focus on how you can continue to make improvements over the coming weeks and months. It is not unusual to worry that sleep will deteriorate on stopping the diaries. It can help to put together a list of all the techniques you have learned and to review the diaries from when you started, to work out what has gone well and what might still be a problem. It is unlikely that everything has gone without a hitch, but hopefully your sleep will have improved significantly. If you try the techniques in this chapter and continue to have difficulties with your sleep, do talk to your doctor.

Some people use technology to help them get a good night's sleep. There are two main types of sleep apps. Some offer a selection of natural sounds – such as water lapping a shore, or rainfall – that aim to induce relaxation and sleepiness. The other type offers a more active, clinically validated course of sleep treatment as described in this chapter and can be accessed directly or prescribed by a doctor. Examples include Sleepstation and Sleepio – see Appendix 3: Resources (for Chapter 4) for more information about sleep apps. But as noted earlier, apps on devices such as phones and watches are generally inaccurate when measuring sleep.

In summary, we now know that sleep has a prominent daily role in maintaining physical and mental health, through the work done by the brain when we are all on a leave of absence overnight! On a 'lighter' note to finish – all the science on improving metabolism through improving sleep would suggest that better sleep will help with weight loss – perhaps not so strange to think we have more chance of sleeping off, rather than running off, those extra pounds.

Key points from Chapter 4

- Try, if you can, to prioritise getting good sleep.

- Sleep is a very active time for metabolism. Healing,

repair, restoration and memory maintenance all occur while we sleep.

• We all sleep and we all wake up several times a night – normally!

• Optimum sleep duration varies and changes with age.

• Insufficient or disrupted sleep increases the risk of developing T2D.

• We are programmed to sleep at night and our systems work best when we sleep at a similar time each day.

• Only natural sleep is beneficial to health.

• Tried and tested tips for improving sleep are widely available, and all *can* help.

• CBT is a proven treatment for insomnia.

Type 2 diabetes: reversal and remission

FAST – food and eating part 1

Remission of T2D – effectively being T2D-free long-term – is a fairly recent concept, and brings into play a tantalising new aiming point and a completely different strategy for managing T2D. It cannot be achieved by medication – only by a change in lifestyle. In other words, only by you!

The possibility of reversing the chemistry of T2D came initially from the results of people having weight loss (bariatric) surgery. Not only did people lose a great deal of weight, but related problems like T2D or high blood pressure simply disappeared, with more than half of people able to continue disease-free for many years.

Before this, once T2D developed, it was always regarded as being permanent. Standard dietary advice for weight loss more often than not failed to give lasting results, and medical treatment of raised blood glucose and increasingly raised blood pressure became 'the treatment' for T2D.

We understand better now that the complications of T2D are not all down to poor control or bad luck – they are part and parcel of the disease. They happen less if glucose and blood pressure are well managed – but they still happen. Medical treatment lowers the risk of T2D complications modestly, but the disease is still there, doing what it does.

Weight loss surgery showed that dramatically reducing food energy going into the body cleared the liver fat which was looking like a major factor in how T2D came about. Doctors then focused on achieving the same outcome using *very* low-calorie diets. Surgery without the surgery approach! Sure enough, similar results were seen, not quite so dramatically perhaps, but without the drama and drawbacks of surgery. Most people lost enough weight and reversed their T2D.

Meanwhile, others were testing whether carbohydrate restriction would do the same thing, arguing that if blood glucose was too high, why feed it? Carbohydrate excess was seen to be the main driver of the damaging liver fat preceding T2D. The results were surprisingly similar, given that very low-carb diets limit carbohydrate intake only, with no overall calorie restriction.

Some people have always known that T2D can be put into remission by dietary means – those who achieved it themselves, usually after a major life change with big weight loss. Long-term studies, too, have shown a very small number of people spontaneously going into remission of their T2D; observations which have shown that reversing T2D, for an individual person, *can happen.*

But there is now good research showing that two dietary changes and surgery can, for very many people, reverse T2D – a disease we thought was *for life* – and there is a groundswell of people in many countries who are gearing up for this challenging new possibility!

The terms 'remission' and 'reversal' have both been used in the last few years. Reversal describes what's happening in the body when T2D is being turned round – and the methods used to do that. Remission is the ongoing absence of T2D – the aiming point and the start of your life journey without T2D. There will still be an even bigger job to do though: remaining T2D-free.

What's involved in getting T2D into remission?

If you managed to hang on in through Chapter 2, you'll be aware that things have had to go very wrong – especially in your liver – for T2D to come about. So you will know that things have to go very *right* to reverse those changes, and that what you do to make that happen needs to continue long-term.

Turning energy right down! Drastically lowering the intake of food energy and available carbohydrate means the body needs a replacement source of fuel – quickly. Liver fat is the most readily available and, as it happens, is the key to unlocking T2D. Reducing liver fat and lowering glucose going into the body is like opening a pressure valve on the liver, which can recover some of its insulin sensitivity, which in turn helps blood glucose to drop further. Lower glucose means less chance of turning more back into liver fat, and the liver can stay unclogged.

A less fatty liver means less fat to release into the bloodstream, allowing it to clear from sites in the body where it should never have been in the first place – notably the pancreas. Insulin production, which may have been dropping, now has a chance to recover long-term – so long as the liver fat doesn't return!

T2D usually develops over many years, typically with slow weight gain and steadily rising insulin, insulin resistance and glucose levels. Once the liver takes on too much fat, the process speeds up, perhaps over one or two years.

When T2D can be reversed, the reduction in liver fat to get the process going is much quicker – days to weeks – and the body loses its excess visible fat over a few months.

As T2D develops, when we gain weight, the liver is the last place to take up extra fat.

As T2D disappears, the liver is the first place to lose fat, before general weight loss occurs.

So we start to get healthier before we get thinner! A process which has been building over months to years can take just a week to *start* turning around. Clearing excess fat – especially from the pancreas – and returning insulin levels to normal, will take much longer, if it can still happen.

Figure 5.1: T2D in reverse gear

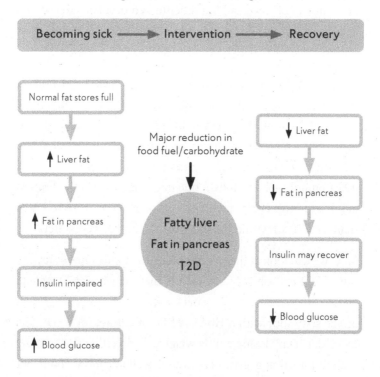

When fuel from food (glucose) drops, by dietary or surgical means, the liver gives up its fat (right side of Figure 5.1), which is now needed by the body for energy, and stops making new fat; so less fat leaving the liver allows it to clear from other places, notably the pancreas. As fat slowly clears from the pancreas, insulin secretion has a good chance of recovering, though that can't be guaranteed. If insulin function is restored (and the liver's owner can avoid re-filling it with fat) the T2D will stay in remission. This is T2D reversal in action and the beginning of normal order being restored!

Improved insulin function doesn't just allow blood glucose to normalise (T2D reversal) but other linked problems to recover. Less insulin resistance means lower blood pressure and, most importantly, a lower risk of artery disease (see Chapter 7).

But getting beyond immediate reversal, what's the definition of remission of T2D? The latest international definition is that HbA1c should be less than 48mmol/mol (6.5%) for at least three months, with no ongoing diabetes medication. Remember that normal is less than 42mmol/mol (6.0%), and 42–48mmol/mol is 'at risk' but not diabetic. This definition is a beginning. For remission to be permanent, HbA1c lower than 42 (6.0%) within the first year would be even better.

Now we can look at the two main dietary approaches to reversing T2D. Firstly, a very low-calorie diet, which was Margaret's choice. To refresh on Margaret's journey, she was diagnosed at age sixty-four with a HbA1c of 60mmol/mol, or 7.6%. She tackled T2D by losing a little weight, then getting fit – playing badminton, doing gym classes and walking more. Both her weight and HbA1c improved, but then came a problem. She injured a knee ligament which stopped her exercising properly and then lost momentum with her diet, such that over a few months, her weight and HbA1c slowly started to rise.

After a conversation with her diabetes nurse, with her husband present, Margaret decided to see if she could get her T2D into remission. Her husband acknowledged that he too could do with losing a few pounds and recognised that if they tackled it together it would be more likely to succeed for his wife.

T2D reversal

1. A short-term, very low-calorie diet. After seeing the diabetes dietician, Margaret and her husband Terry invested in a two-month liquid meal-replacement plan – three 200kcal drinks per day with another 200kcal made up from roughage (mixed greens, to help prevent constipation and keep them chewing). The vitamin-fortified drinks were available in different flavours and their cost was offset by having almost no food shopping for eight weeks!

(Note: to avoid confusion, 'calories' in common language around nutrition and diets is actually scientifically the kilocalorie and appears on food labels as kcals. The metric equivalent is the kilojoule or kJ. One kilocalorie = 4.2 kilojoules.)

So, what is a very low-calorie diet? It's one that delivers just 800kcal or less per day. In other words, only about a third of normal daily energy use, and not much more than the brain itself uses each day to keep everything running. No wonder people call this a starvation diet!

But don't worry, a body with T2D has all the stored energy needed to manage – we can last for two or three months on a lifeboat without food, so 800kcal a day for the same amount of time is no problem. Two or three months is usually what's needed for this first phase, which is designed to pull fat from the liver and improve insulin function.

Experts reckon that losing at least 10kg, ideally 15kg (22–33lb), makes T2D reversal more likely. If you weigh much less than 80kg, then around 15 per cent of your weight lost should be enough, which could be as little as 10kg (22lb).

Why not eat real food – and why go so fast? There's no reason why real food cannot be used for this – there are many liquid meal and pre-prepared food alternatives available commercially to suit all types of diet (see chapter resources in Appendix 3). You can make your own if you have sufficient time, enthusiasm and calorie-management skills (or a very helpful dietician). If you want to save money, four 500ml drinks of skimmed milk per day with a multivitamin and some roughage will do the job at a fraction of the cost!

A weight loss of 15kg (33lb) can reverse T2D, whether it takes two months or two years, but with this rapid approach it's much more likely to hit that target, and reduce the chances of a person quitting.

The result: Margaret and Terry supported each other to lose 27kg – almost 60lb – between them in about ten weeks. Margaret lost 13kg and her blood glucose and blood pressure became normal without medication. Three months into the diet, after replacing some of the drinks with small real-food meals, Margaret started to regain weight. She felt her resolve slip after a couple of meals out with alcohol. Margaret and Terry went back to replacement drinks for a further two weeks, which helped Margaret to stabilise her weight. In the months afterwards, she stayed off alcohol, and weight gain was minimal. Her T2D remission held over the following months as food and calories slowly increased. We'll join the couple again in the next chapter, when we look at their options for keeping it all going after this first weight loss phase. Margaret and Terry had a plan for potential 'relapse', involving having support on hand and managing their alcohol consumption. The value of support when trying to reverse T2D cannot be overstated.

How well does the very low-calorie phase work? Overall, using this approach, an impressive 50 per cent or more of people have managed to be T2D-free at one year. Remission occurred in the large majority of people who achieved and maintained 15kg or more of weight loss, and in about half of those with 10–15kg weight loss.

What's good about it?

- It works quickly and rapid weight loss helps build motivation.

- Hunger and lethargy occur – but are less than might be expected.

- It's not complicated, especially with replacement drinks or food plans.

What's not so good?

- Once weight loss is under way, it's common to feel cold, as the body adjusts its internal thermostat to save energy.

- Mild temporary hair shedding can occur – but it always recovers.

- The gradual adjustment to more normal eating, while still holding calories lower than previously, is *much* the hardest part.

This diet would usually be done with support from a diabetes dietician or a clinician with suitable nutritional expertise. A multivitamin is needed if using real food (food-replacement drinks are usually supplemented), and almost everyone needs fibre/roughage (occasionally medication) to help prevent constipation. Stopping or reducing medication for T2D and blood pressure is usual at the outset, so monitoring is essential.

More information on very low-calorie eating, including links to non-dairy options, for this phase are in Appendix 3: Resources (for Chapter 5) – signposting Professor Roy Taylor's book *Life Without Diabetes*, which explains T2D reversal and very low-calorie eating in some depth – highly recommended.

2. Low-carbohydrate eating. If you have read up on weight loss, you might have come across the abbreviation LCD – low-carbohydrate (low-carb) diet. Although it feels fairly recent, low-carb eating is not actually new – in fact, it goes way back. Around one hundred and fifty years ago, medical authorities acknowledged that starchy foods (carbohydrates) needed to be 'taken in moderation' for weight and health. Before the arrival of insulin in the 1920s, when there was no formal recognition of the different types of diabetes, *everyone* was managed with a very low-carbohydrate diet. This kept people with type 1 diabetes alive a little longer, and may have put some people with T2D into remission – we don't know. The recent rise in the disease, and a focus on insulin and insulin resistance has stimulated interest in low-carbohydrate approaches in T2D around the world.

Glucose from carbohydrates is the main trigger for insulin release. Lowering carbohydrate intake lowers insulin levels and improves insulin resistance, which improves the way the body handles both glucose and fat (see Chapter 2). Over a century after it was the only treatment for diabetes, low-carbohydrate eating is now recognised internationally as a way of improving T2D and a legitimate route to remission. Such are the ebbs and flows of nutritional advice!

What is low carbohydrate? There will be more on nutrient groups and foods in the next chapter and the resources, but here's a reminder: the common carb-rich foods are potatoes, pasta, rice, bread and all sugary things – biscuits and cakes, confectionery, sweetened drinks and many fruits. Baked goods are generally rich in both carbohydrate and fat. When did you last have a day with little or none of these foods?

Low-carb eating might seem like a simple matter of eating less of the above – and is probably good advice for everyone – especially if we include packaged processed foods, which are notorious for added sugars. But if your aim is T2D remission, something more structured is needed.

To give a feel for how dietary carb intake is labelled, Table 5.1 shows the accepted guidance (TDE is total daily energy as calories).

Table 5.1: Carbohydrate calories per day

Carbohydrate (diet)	Carbohydrate (amount)	Energy from Carbohydrate	Proportion of TDE
Very Low	< 50g/day	< 200 kcal/day	< 10%
Low	< 130g/day	< 520 kcal/day	< 26%
Intermediate	< 225g/day	< 900 kcal/day	< 45%
High	> 225g/day	> 900 kcal/day	> 45%

The figures are based on a notional 2,000kcal/day, the recommended amount to avoid weight gain (this is less than most people eat currently).

Around the world, nutritional guidance – and it varies a little – is for carbs to make up between just under a half to around two-thirds of total daily energy intake. If you are used to eating as much as 60 per cent of your calories or more as carbohydrate, lowering that to 10 per cent (a *very* low-carb diet) will feel quite challenging. In terms of the impact on metabolism and T2D, this is the equivalent of a very low-calorie diet or bariatric surgery.

To reverse T2D, a *very* low-carb diet of less than 50g per day works best of all, but the lower you go, the harder it can feel to adapt to life without foods which we now take for granted. A 'regular' low-carbohydrate diet – officially less than 130g per day and ideally less than 100g per day – can also work reasonably well and be easier to live with. A practical approach would be to eat very low carb for two to four months, then relax the restriction slowly, to feel for the point, if any, at which weight and/or (reversed) T2D begin to return.

What does 50g of carbohydrate look like?

- Three small slices of bread.

- A small/average portion of pasta or rice.

- Three small potatoes.

This would be your *daily* limit for these foods. By contrast, you could have a very large plate of salad or vegetables, over 200g (almost half a pound) of mixed nuts and even more berries for your 50g and still be in business!

Most typical main meals contain more than 50g of carbohydrate. The spaghetti bolognese we used for reference in Chapter 2 would get you to about 100g in a single meal, so eating pasta, potatoes or bread is a challenge when aiming low.

Can we manage with no carbohydrate at all? Well, in theory yes – there are no essential carbohydrates (unlike protein and fats) and the liver can make all the glucose we need, but going as low as zero is impractical and not necessary.

Indigenous peoples who eat virtually no carbs, such as the

Maasai of East Africa, have no health consequences from their largely fat- and protein-based diets. They are adapted, which is important when eating with minimal carbs. The body 'learns' to run on fat, which becomes its main fuel.

But how can we feed the brain? If the brain needs 600kcal of energy a day, and only (usually) runs on glucose, that's about 150g – so 50g is very low. The brain adapts to a very low carb intake by running partly on glucose made in the liver, and partly on ketones which our liver makes from fat. We are evolved to use ketones in times of fast and famine – they even seem to sharpen up our brain! So our 50g per day very low-carb diet is actually very safe (*and* we can do puzzles faster!).

There's more on ketones and low-carb eating in Chapter 6, but for now let's just say that it's really effective for improving and reversing T2D. To begin with, it is complex and easy to get wrong, and most definitely needs the guidance of a dietician or doctor who is familiar with the approach.

So how well does it work for T2D? It produces weight loss, and improvements in blood glucose and insulin, at least on a par with very low-calorie diets – though it has to be said that major research programmes of both are not well matched for making comparisons. Your chance of putting T2D into remission improves as you lower your carb intake, and depends on whether you can sustain and adapt to this way of eating long-term. Research in a primary care (non-specialist) setting, has shown that this is highly achievable.

What's good about it?

- Again – it works!

- When eating low carb, there is no need to consciously restrict calories – cutting out most carbohydrate is enough to favourably impact T2D.

- Hunger is not usually an issue at any stage, and being able to eat non-carb food freely means that energy balance can be left to the body to sort out!

- Studies show that, when adapted (which takes about three or four weeks), most people naturally eat less than they did, without calorie-counting, and energy levels are reported to be good.

- This sounds so good, why would we advocate any other method?! Nothing is perfect.

What's not so good?

- It's a little more complex than you might think – a good guide/support is so important. Lowering or stopping T2D and blood pressure medication will be needed.

- A low-carb diet, perhaps from lowering insulin, causes the kidneys to excrete more sodium (salt) and water, which can cause faintness, fatigue and cramps. You may need extra salt, running against usual advice.

- 'Fat fear' – see below.

- We have lived in a world dominated by carbohydrate for decades now, so the switch away from this nutrient group is challenging at home, when shopping and when eating out. Be prepared.

Low-carb (especially *very* low-carb) eating means eating more fat – going against prevailing official nutritional advice, the view of your own doctor or nurse, and quite possibly your own beliefs, as low-fat has been the dominant theme in nutrition for almost half a century. We hope the section on fat fear in the next chapter will help, but remember – carbohydrates drive up insulin naturally and we are looking to get insulin down to help with insulin resistance. Eating too much carbohydrate is the main driver of fatty liver, and related insulin resistance. It may feel like an act of faith to eat this way, but seeing blood tests and blood pressure readings improving will help overcome a lot of the uncertainty.

Low-carb eating (especially very low) takes some learning and/ or guidance, and finding a good guide may not always be easy. It also takes time to adapt – try to give it at least four to six weeks before judging how you feel and whether progress is being made.

Anyone can try low-carb eating, but if you live and eat with others, it's important to have their support, even if they're not doing exactly the same themselves. Low-carb eating is both short- and long-term in terms of T2D reversal, and therefore remission, and eating long-term to preserve good health; more on this in Chapter 6.

After a similar initial success using the same approach as Margaret (low-calorie eating), Colin struggled with some distracting hunger and switched to a low-carbohydrate diet which he found surprisingly easy, and his hunger issue settled within two weeks of making the switch.

Timing a dietary change

This is a very personal decision. The first phase of trying to put T2D into remission, with a substantial change or reduction in eating, is going to take at least two or three months. Christmas (or any major holiday event) might be best avoided, but some people disagree. Preparation should include a discussion with friends and family – they will want to be supportive, and it's helpful for people to know you need to be strict with food for some time to come. At home, think about a kitchen cupboard and shopping plan, depending on your choice of diet.

It's probably best to write down some initial targets for weight and blood glucose, and most importantly, to discuss with your healthcare team what to do about a possible lack of progress or weight gain. How much would trigger a response, and what should the response be? Margaret went back on to replacement drinks after gaining 3kg (7lb) and got things back under control. Planning ahead means a thoughtful response to slippage can be quickly implemented.

3. Bariatric surgery. Bariatric or weight loss surgery has been known for many years to impact on T2D. This approach has been gathering momentum around the world over the past decade, such that some people are starting to call it 'metabolic surgery' – surgery that alters metabolism! Surgery has taught doctors a great deal about digestion and energy metabolism, and it became a springboard for dietary reversal of T2D in recent years.

Surgery works on many levels – it's not just shrinking the stomach! It reduces the capacity for food to be taken in, and for most procedures it reduces the digestion and absorption of nutrients.

Some types of surgery have complex effects on the body, involving the chemistry and bacteria in the intestine (the microbiome) and the wider hormone system of the body. It's fair to say that understanding what happens in surgical 're-plumbing' of the human gut is still in its infancy.

The first week of enforced rest for the stomach after surgery, and the need for quick energy, allows a relieved liver to give up some of its accumulated fat. Losing liver fat immediately improves insulin function and blood glucose drops quickly – well before weight loss becomes noticeable. Surgery was originally intended to help people with major weight and weight-related health problems. If you have a BMI over 40, you are likely to be eligible, if it's available where you live, whether you have T2D or not. You may be eligible with a BMI of 35 or even 30 if you have T2D. As a guide:

An average height man: BMI 40 = 121kg (266lb)
BMI 35 = 107kg (235lb)
An average height woman: BMI 40 = 108kg (238lb)
BMI 35 = 95kg (210lb)

What are the results for T2D remission? Average weight loss exceeds 40kg (88lb) – around a third of total body weight – at one year. About two-thirds of people can go into remission from T2D in the year after bariatric surgery, with a large proportion of people maintaining that over many years.

What's good about it?

- Weight loss is assured and remission of T2D is very likely.

- Reduced fatty liver, blood pressure and risk of heart attack and stroke.

- Some people report improvements in self-esteem and confidence from major weight loss.

- Where surgery is available there are likely to be health-care system savings.

What's not good?

- Surgery comes with risks – these risks are generally low considering the challenge of operating on large people, but occasionally they can be serious.

- Long-term medical supervision is needed to monitor for nutritional deficiencies, and to support and advise those who struggle with an enforced new eating pattern.

- Dumping syndrome – see below.

The phenomenon known as 'dumping syndrome' is the most reported and troublesome long-term physical complication of surgery. Unnaturally rapid emptying of concentrated stomach contents can produce abdominal cramps, diarrhoea, sweating, flushing and nausea soon after eating. It can be eased by dietary adjustments, but can be stubborn to manage, and some people describe post-surgical life as 'juggling with dumping syndrome'.

Psychosocial aspects of bariatric surgery. There is a strong case for psychological support before and long-term after bariatric surgery. Many people – especially women – who have this surgery are depressed, and this may not resolve afterwards. Changes in body size and shape are experienced personally, and redundant skin after major weight loss is not a trivial issue. Obesity and T2D are both highly complex, and bariatric surgery itself does some very complex things to the human body, so unsurprisingly the experience of living long-term with what some have called the 'bariatric body' can be uncertain.

Bariatric surgery can look great from a doctor's perspective, but it must be lived with. We would urge people with T2D who are considering bariatric surgery to weigh up the long-term issues, and to read and talk to people who have had surgery. Some procedures are irreversible or tricky to re-do. You should expect to receive long-term medical supervision after surgery – if that doesn't happen, raise it with your healthcare team.

Both UK and international bariatric surgery registries confirm the very strong connections between weight, T2D, high blood pressure, depression and obstructive sleep apnoea (as discussed in Chapter 4). But in general only around one in a hundred potentially eligible people undergo surgery for obesity and related problems. There are simply too many people with T2D, let alone obesity, for surgery to be a realistic solution; and in any event it just seems the wrong way to tackle a preventable medical problem. Improved medical (nutritional) management of T2D is here with us, and can only get better.

Summary of the three main approaches to reversing T2D

Bariatric or metabolic surgery works well for weight loss and T2D, but with complex effects on the body and how people feel about themselves – both good and bad. It needs careful thought and additional psychological support.

Low-calorie or low-carbohydrate eating can be tried by anyone, with healthcare support. Most doctors will advocate stopping or lowering medication selectively, for both T2D and blood pressure, from whenever the change is made.

But what else might work? Some years ago, when a group of middle-aged Australian Aboriginal people with T2D reverted to their traditional hunter-gatherer (HG) lifestyle for just seven weeks, all of the metabolic abnormalities of diabetes were greatly improved or reversed. Conversely, when any small-scale Indigenous society transitions to a larger, modern, industrialised one, then weight gain, high blood pressure, artery disease and T2D appear. The main differences in lifestyle that might impact on metabolic health are worth mentioning, since the experience of disease is so radically different in the two settings.

HG diets are typically lower in energy but with no particular standout macronutrient pattern – though they are mostly higher in protein and lower in carbohydrate than typical modern diets. They show a wide diversity of natural wholefoods and a much higher intake of fibre.

As we've already said, HG populations are significantly more active than we are. But in spite of this, they do not use more energy overall than we do. Being active hasn't made them lean, though it probably keeps them so; it does help them to stay healthy.

HG communities spend much more time outdoors in fresh air. Low levels of stress and mental health problems may relate to a more cohesive community life – with strong family bonds and low levels of inequality. We can't become hunter-gatherers but we can condense some of their lifestyle lessons into thinking about more options for reversing T2D, overlapping with our FAST suggestion.

Food – eating a wide variety of natural foods, which will tend to be less energy-dense, but more nutrient-rich, and have more fibre, such as the Mediterranean diet. Hunter-gatherers don't eat processed foods! (See Chapter 6.)

Be as active as you can – or do as much exercise as you feel able to. It will give you the best chance of reversing T2D

(Chapter 3), but again, bear in mind that in the early weeks of a very low-calorie or low-carbohydrate diet stick to moderate exercise like regular walks until transitional fatigue settles.

Sleep in tune with nature – HGs are said to have similar basic sleep patterns and durations to those of us who sleep well. Insomnia is a rare occurrence and cooler ambient temperatures help their sleep, reinforcing the general advice for us all to keep our bedrooms cool.

Deal with stress – any significant mental health problem drives the link between the brain and the body's stress hormone, cortisol, which worsens insulin resistance, increasing the risk of T2D and artery disease. HG communities are relatively cohesive and equitable, with low reported levels of stress and mental illness.

All of these have a bearing on insulin resistance, and taking positive action in all areas might together be enough to help reverse T2D. Another dietary option would be to **cut out sugar**. A low-carbohydrate diet can reverse T2D. But what if we just took a part of our carbohydrate intake away – the part that is sugar. Might that work too? Sugar (fructose) consumption has been rising in recent times along with T2D and expert opinion is growing on the potential role of fructose in T2D and other metabolic disease.

Compelling clinical research shows that eliminating fructose in the diet can reverse abnormalities in liver fat, insulin and glucose. Might it reverse full-on T2D too? We don't know for sure, but it's worth bearing in mind that fructose has no known health benefits, so eliminating it would appear to be a risk-free strategy in tackling T2D. We'll look in more detail at dietary fructose, and the confusing terminology around 'sugar' in Chapter 6.

Eat differently and work harder in the gym – eating fewer times a day, fasting in its various forms and high-intensity exercise all have their supporters in terms of improving, even reversing, T2D. No reason not to consider any or all of these things. Just because large-scale, controlled trials have not been done, it doesn't mean they won't work – there is decent science underpinning all of them (see next chapter).

If (when!) my T2D is in remission, do I still need medical check-ups?

Yes, definitely! We don't yet know whether reversal or remission will immediately lower the risk of T2D complications, so monitoring your circulation, eyes, kidneys and so forth needs to continue for the time being. If you have diabetic eye disease you will need specialist advice before attempting reversal, as a sudden lowering of blood glucose may occasionally make your eyes worse before they get better.

We think the risks connected with T2D will lower quickly after reversal but might take longer to return fully to the level of a person without T2D – but that should happen if you keep it up.

We'll leave you to think about T2D remission around these three thoughts:

1. Reversal works – remission is achievable!

Firstly, T2D *can* be reversed and put into remission. The best time to try is soon after diagnosis – remember T2D will have been with you for a while, even years, but psychologically it's a fresh blow, so don't give it time to take root in your mind. Hit back as soon as you can! Even better if your tests show that you are at risk of T2D but do not yet have it – reversing 'at risk' is potentially easier, as Suzanne did initially (and Alan needed to try!).

It's *possible* that anyone can do it, but you have to be aware that the chances are lower the longer you've had the disease. The reasons why things don't start working again are complex, and may be out of your hands (genes again!). But people *have* managed, even after twenty years – and you will never know if you don't try!

Whichever route you choose involves a big change in eating and a new relationship with food, so you will need to carefully weigh up what's involved both short- and long-term before you can decide what's best for you.

Ted decided not to explore the option of reversal. He had minor symptoms and felt that, at the age of seventy-eight, it was not worth such a big change in his (and his wife's) way of life just to prevent *possible* future problems.

Margaret lost her initial good control of T2D following a knee injury. She was unable to exercise and lost her way a little with her diet. Later she was able to 'regroup' and focus on attempting dietary reversal of her disease.

Everyone's circumstances are different, and age can make the world feel different. Knowing what's involved in remission can help you to choose your path, so do get as much information as you can. The really important thing to know now is that you have a choice.

2. Standard treatment doesn't target T2D itself

You know now that medical treatment has been focused on the raised glucose part of T2D. But having perfect or normal blood glucose is nigh on impossible, and trying too hard to achieve that can bring its own problems, especially when insulin is involved. Changing the way you eat to try to reverse T2D can help a great deal. Even if the disease is still there, it will be much improved – as will your health. And medication, including insulin, can often be avoided.

3. Holding T2D in remission is harder than achieving remission in the first place

So far, research suggests that about half of people getting into remission over a year have lost it again within another year. It's hard to retain 'changed eating' in the kind of world most of us live in, but it's not impossible if you can work on your relationship with food and learn how to live comfortably with changed eating – which is what much of the next chapter is about.

Pause for thought

If you have been diagnosed with T2D, were you aware that T2D could be reversed, or put into remission, by eating changes or weight-loss surgery?

Have you been given information, advice and support about T2D reversal/remission?

Do you know anyone with T2D who has mentioned the topic or tried to achieve it themselves?

If you haven't already done so, try to speak to your nurse or doctor about T2D remission, what's happening where you live, what local resources you can access fairly easily and who you can talk to – this may guide the path for you. Help from a diabetes specialist nurse, a doctor with experience in diabetes and/or ideally a dietician or nutritionist with diabetes experience would all be good.

Reversing T2D is about knowledge and getting the right help, but it's even more about mindset – you will need to be absolutely focused on the job in hand, and you will need buckets of determination to succeed. Casual attention to it won't help. Getting the right help does not mean only professional help, in fact the help of friends, especially family, is almost the most important help and second only to self-help!

Key points from Chapter 5

- T2D can be reversed and put into remission by dietary means.

- Reducing liver fat (and preventing its return) is a key step in the process.

- Very low-calorie or very low-carbohydrate diets are the methods with more evidence but other approaches might work too.

- Remission of T2D is currently held to be a HbA1c value of 48mmol/mol (6.5%) for at least three months with no ongoing diabetes medication.

- Attempting reversal of T2D needs a high level of professional and personal support.

- Holding remission long-term is a bigger challenge than achieving initial reversal.

Eating well for the long haul

FAST – food and eating part 2

Chapter 5 was mainly about the process of reversing T2D, and in this second 'food chapter' we will look at eating to maintain remission of T2D, which is essentially the same as long-term healthy eating! We think there are two main lessons from the early experiences of reversal:

Lesson one is that reversal can work and offers a new option for managing T2D. The disease can be reversed by very low-calorie/carbohydrate diets and by bariatric surgery. It might be possible to reverse T2D by eating a low- or no-sugar diet, or a wholefood diet like the Mediterranean diet. These could work for individuals, but pending further research they are still possibilities, not certainties. Weight loss of 15kg – and maintenance of that lost weight – is likely to clear the liver and pancreas of excess fat, helping restore normal insulin function. Less weight loss may still work in leaner people and with low-carbohydrate diets. Even if the disease is not fully reversed, weight loss can still help greatly with T2D control. Reversing and holding T2D in remission means looking after your liver.

Lesson two is that it takes a big and sustained effort from people to manage T2D in this new way. Those who have successfully navigated their way out of T2D, especially those in longer-term remission, found:

• A deep (inner) **motivation** to make and sustain a changed way of eating.

• **Knowledge** to guide them.

• **Something that worked** – *for them.*

Sometimes finding something that works precedes the other elements. Knowledge *can* be a driver, but the other two elements are ultimately more important, and finding something that works is the overall aim.

EXERCISE

Think about what deep or inner motivation might mean to you

Knowledge can give you a sense of direction but not the purpose to strive on – especially when things get tough. You have to find and hold on to what ultimately really motivates you; you will need to draw on it from time to time. Keep a note of this and share it with someone close to you if you can.

We know from studying the reversal of T2D that motivation, and what that means to an individual, is really important for the long haul. If you have managed to reverse T2D, you will have done something really special. But you cannot rest on your laurels – holding remission over the longer term is much more difficult and your motivation will be tested.

Of our cases, Margaret had the goal of staying well into older age to see her family growing up. Only she knows if this will be enough.

Suzanne never really defined hers – a low-carbohydrate diet worked for her when she was at risk of T2D, and she lost weight. But her motivation really only hardened up when she relapsed and developed T2D. It became more solid again when she learned that her daughter's health had a link to her own (see Chapter 9). Family and long-term wellbeing can be powerful motivators.

Sustainability and what works

Something that works for you is easier to sustain if that change makes you *feel* better in some way. If a benefit is less felt, you have to work harder with motivation to sell the sustainment of change to yourself. It's worth trying to understand what you need from a change to help it stick.

If you stop smoking and get to the point when you can breathe more easily, that might help you not restart more than the long-term factors (the money saved and lower cancer risk).

Writing about T1D, Adam Brown makes the excellent point that finding an eating pattern for good glucose control works for him as it improves his mood, which in turn impacts positively on his relationships. Having better day-to-day life and happier relationships motivates him more than fear of long-term health risks – which he (and perhaps most of us) finds much harder to engage with (see Appendix 4: Further reading for Chapter 8 – self-monitoring).

People who reverse their T2D are two or three times more likely to sustain weight loss and their T2D remission than people who diet to lose weight. Weight regain comes from the struggle with motivation – not an ineffective diet. If motivation can trip us up, it might be worth spending more time thinking this through *before* making a change.

Pause for thought

Reversing or improving T2D means new learning, some hard work and a high level of commitment. We've just asked you to think about what can or does motivate you. Is this something that you might need to work on?

Cassie valued her personal health and fitness most. Adam Brown valued his relationships. Finding something that works and keeping it going needs motivation that is very personal to you.

This chapter is about food and eating, but at every turn of the T2D journey remember FAST: being active is better at helping maintain weight loss than achieving it, and attend to any issues around sleep and stress. All will increase the chance of staying well over time.

Before we look at long-term dietary options, we want to mention a few things on dietary research and weight loss which we think are relevant to T2D. Firstly, research confirms just how hard achieving long-term weight loss can be – unhelpful and unhealthy cycles of on/off dieting with up and down weight have characterised the rise in obesity (and weight loss attempts) in the last few decades. Everyone tends to lose weight initially when they diet but with a large variation between people and between diets, so clearly some approaches work better for some individuals.

Secondly, most people (but not everyone) regain their lost weight, over months or longer. Some weight regain is from adjustments in the body's autopilot, but mostly it's that we drift back to the habits and behaviours which made us gain weight in the first place. In other words, we didn't *sustain* our new eating pattern.

If we can maintain an approach that works it will usually continue to work. This is helpful to know in T2D, where a way of eating which works for you has to be for life.

EXERCISE

Why do you think most people don't sustain an eating change long-term? And why, if this applied to you in the past, did you not stick to your plan(s)? Don't worry – you're not alone!

Compare your thoughts with ones we've collected, but go with what's important to *you*:

- 'I was bored and just missed some foods'

- 'The diet didn't fit my personal lifestyle or work'

- 'It was awkward fitting in with friends and family'

- 'I was always craving certain foods'

- 'The foods I like are the things I shouldn't have been eating – but I was'

- 'I was always hungry'

- 'I found shops too full of temptations'

- 'Snacking helped my mood and stress'

Diet failure is a mixed bag, and overeating is caused by different things. The biggest struggles are probably eating to relieve tension or low mood, and actual hunger. Hunger comes to us from different directions. In biology, hunger is nature's way of telling us we are short of readily available food energy – some call this somatic hunger – a real bodily sensation. But sometimes we find ourselves browsing our cupboards when we have time on our hands – we're looking for something to do, or sitting at a screen all day, and snacking is pleasurable. Some call this 'boredom eating' or 'habit grazing' and it helps to understand the difference and your own patterns.

We'll ask you to complete a food diary shortly which can help you to think about what you do. Snacking is a major reason why diets fail. Understanding why some diets make this worse can be helpful.

We can dissipate or distract hunger. Have you ever worked a long shift or been diverted from your routines for a full day, without food? Hunger doesn't always come, or maybe goes unnoticed.

Being mentally active and/or physically occupied are important for managing mood but also for containing and training physical sensations like hunger, and to counter a 'grazing' mentality.

Healthy eating and you. For a moment, forget theories and the generality of it all and focus on yourself. The aim of healthy eating is not to *stick* to a diet or follow an eating guideline – it's to be healthy. If you have T2D or are at risk of it, *you* are unwell – and really, the only thing that matters to you is *your* health.

Regardless of whether you have been following trusted advice, or just feel that you are eating well, if you have T2D, then by definition your eating is out of tune with the needs of your body. You now have to find a way of eating that is in tune with those needs.

Pause for thought

Towards the end of Chapter 1, we asked you to
reflect on your own weight gain, to get a sense
of when and how this happened. Revisit that
information, or work it out now if you passed on it
before. Thinking about when T2D might have started
could help you to get a sense of *how* it started.

Let's define healthy eating in the way that we defined good
sleep. Let's relate healthy eating to health rather than advice or
a guideline. Healthy eating is what you are doing when you are
free of disease and feel well, with a good sense of energy. You
will have a healthy liver – free of excess fat – and stable weight.

This definition, which targets health, is a much simpler starting point than one which starts with a theory around nutrients
or food. It follows from this that individual variation is accept-
able and it gives us permission to experiment when things are
not going well.

In a T2D context, a healthy diet is the one that works! When
eating healthily, HbA1c will be normal, as will blood pressure,
ideally without medication. Without scanning, none of us
can know for sure if we have normal liver fat or not, and in
the near future tests will offer up a simpler way of assessing
healthy metabolism. But for now, weight and waistline will
guide, and a normal liver blood test can reassure.

T2D and having permission to change. This may be a time for you to think about what has happened (or not happened perhaps) in your life for you to be where you are now. Getting away from T2D is like getting off a slowly sinking ship. The first step on the lifeboat is getting your diet working for you, ideally to reverse or much improve the disease. Getting properly on to the lifeboat is using that diet or something else which works to keep you safe. After reversing T2D, going back to eating as you were will almost certainly see it return. Give *yourself* permission to change.

EXERCISE

At this point it would be useful to do a food diary which can complement some of your reading and be a good introduction to self-monitoring (Chapter 8).

Ideally, take a look first at what you eat now, using a food diary. Keep it really simple – something like this will do to begin with:

Table 6.1: Food Diary – 7 Days (example of two days)

	Monday	Tuesday
Breakfast	Coffee – sugar 1 Muesli cereal – milk Toast (white) x 2, jam/jelly, orange juice	Coffee – sugar 1 Porridge – milk Bagel, peanut butter

Morning snack	Banana	Fruit yoghurt (shop-bought)
Lunch	Cheese/pickle sandwich – brown Packet crisps/chips Tea – sugar 1	Lasagne – leftover (homemade), coleslaw
Afternoon snack	Biscuits/cookies 2 Tea – sugar 1	Mixed nuts/dried fruit Tea – sugar 1
Tea/ Dinner	Fish/sauce (ready meal), mashed potato/greens	Veg bolognese (homemade) Spaghetti Plain yoghurt/ berries
Evening snack	Decaf tea – sugar 1 Toast (brown) 1 slice	Decaf tea – sugar 1 Biscuits/cookies 2

The example shows just two days but yours will need to cover at least a full week. A blank version as a guide is in Appendix 3: Resources (for Chapter 6).

You don't need to count calories or weigh things to get a general idea of your diet. Use an app if you prefer – anything to be able to see what kind of food you are eating each day, how many meals, snacks and drinks other than plain water. Do this on a typical week or two if you can. Record whether food was homemade (made from scratch) or something you bought (pre-packaged). We'll use that part later.

A food diary, however you do it, has one major benefit – it tells you what you *are* eating, as opposed to what you *think* you are eating. For it to be helpful it has to be complete and truthful – this is for you, remember. It's the beginning of understanding your food choices and patterns of eating. It can be used for discussions with your healthcare practitioner or dietician.

Keep your first week's diary (two weeks if you can). We can look at it again towards the end of the chapter, and again in Chapter 8 when we look at self-monitoring.

Healthy eating for life

The nutritional landscape of T2D has become more complex over the last twenty years and it would take a very large book to cover all the relevant changes around diet alone. So what we are going to do is to highlight first some areas and specific points of interest, controversy and consensus. We are then going to look at the principles of low-calorie and low-carbo-hydrate eating in T2D – along with connected variations such as fasting. We'll conclude by looking at a wholefood dietary approach, using the Mediterranean diet as an example.

We still live with the repercussions of dietary advice which came from the US in 1977. The core of that guidance is to eat less fat, control our calories and portions, keep protein moder-ate, eat plenty of carbohydrates based on more grains and less sugars – and aim for a balance of nutrients.

Restricting dietary fat to provide no more than 30 per cent of total energy overall paved the way for a rise in carbohydrate intake. To follow the nutritional guidelines in the UK, US, Europe or Australia, for example, would mean that two-thirds of food energy will come from (starchy) carbohydrates.

Standard nutritional advice has relaxed a little in terms of over-all fat intake, but still advocates restricting saturated fat to a maximum of 10 per cent of total calories. Dietary fat restriction and advice to eat plentiful carbohydrates remain contentious, though recent official acceptance of reduced carbohydrate eating (and higher fat therefore) suggests that a rethink is coming. There is *so* much more metabolic disease since standard advice was changed. We can't be sure whether the advice is funda-mentally flawed or that too few have followed it, but sharply rising disease suggests that very high levels of carbohydrate simply cannot be good for T2D.

Better understanding of how T2D comes about, and how complex energy use is in the body, are reshaping the way that we view energy balance. Exercise clearly does more than burn calories – its impact on health is greater than that on weight management. Adjusting the calories that we eat is also a more complex business than we once thought.

We know that dietary guidelines may be far removed from what people actually eat. In our own country, awareness of nutritional guidance detail is quite poor, even amongst profes-sionals. In John's clinics, and anecdotally others, carbohydrate intake was often above two-thirds of calorie intake in people with newly diagnosed T2D. Food diaries are essential tools in helping people navigate away from pre-diagnosis eating patterns. Nutritional surveys confirm that we are eating less fat than we did a generation ago but sugar intakes are still too high.

There is recognition that more healthy eating might be more expensive and not always accessible, especially in low-income countries, where T2D and obesity are being driven harder by economic change, with a rise in 'fast food' consumption and the marketing of processed foods, which impacts adversely on more traditional diets. Awareness of barriers to healthy eating is needed, but solutions are clearly not simple.

There is consensus that eating well for all of us is much the same as eating well to both prevent and manage T2D. A 'diabetic diet' therefore is no longer recognised. Within that principle, dietary detail needs to be individualised and there is no one size fits all.

Although food and eating are paramount in managing T2D, people everywhere recognise the importance of being active, sleeping well and managing stress (FAST). Nutritional vocabulary seems to be settling around foods rather than individual nutrients. Which oils are better for us? Are nuts right for T2D? Dairy foods are a leading food group for debate – their value as a food group in T2D is seemingly at odds with their saturated fat content, but such paradoxes are now enriching the debate about healthy eating and maybe whether saturated fat is so bad for us after all. There is good consensus amongst scientists and clinicians that wholefood diets and home cooking are good for T2D, but highly processed foods as a group are not good.

A word of caution on dietary guidance everywhere: we all know – though it's not always stated – that the food industry influences dietary guidance. Our own Eatwell Guide in the UK was produced by a group with strong industry ties. There are many examples of both subtle and more muscular manipulation of political and public opinion to benefit commercial interest. Read Susan Greenhalgh's excellent article on how China aligned with Coca-Cola's position that exercise, not nutrition, was the key to fighting obesity (Appendix 4: Further reading (for Chapter 6). Market economies mean that we should maintain a healthy scepticism on the probity of nutritional guidance.

These things tell us that nothing is set in stone. Diets should be viewed as options or possibilities, and one individual's healthy diet might be a little different to someone else's. Experts emphasise that, above all, we need to sustain any change for it to really work, so as we said before, inner motivation is so important along with what works – which is coming next.

Low-calorie eating

The very low calorie levels which reverse T2D (down to 800kcal per day) can't be sustained beyond a few weeks. In reversal trials, people gradually adjusted to more normal eating, trying to keep to around three-quarters of the calories they had previously consumed. The question of how much cutting back is needed – what works and what's sustainable – has no easy answer. Some people have managed long-term restriction in the 1,200–2,000kcal range (several hundred calories fewer than usually needed), maintaining weight loss, health and staying in control. But most people struggle.

The long-term challenges of daily energy restriction are now well known, as most dieters can testify. Automatic adjustments in eating, of 'felt' energy levels and hunger can all work against us, causing weight regain.

Very low-calorie eating may well be the most effective dietary way to achieve remission of T2D, but it's the hardest way to maintain it. Whether enough people can retain remission (or keep good long-term control) of T2D this way remains to be seen.

In summary, energy restriction – eating less – has some built-in obstacles to sustainability and needs some teeth-gritting, which means that we think this to be a challenging approach for T2D long-term.

Margaret, on a very low-calorie diet, achieved reversal then 'wobbled' (hunger). She got back into remission but, a year later and still on a low-calorie diet, lost full remission. She did, however, stay in good control on minimal medication.

Fasting

A different way of restricting calories which some find more sustainable is intermittent fasting. So far, results are favourable – at least sufficiently favourable to be included in our review of options for T2D.

There are three common variations and, in ascending order of challenge (and probably of effectiveness), they are:

Time-restricted eating. This means limiting the time window of eating each day, for example to twelve, eight, six or even four hours per day. This lengthens the overnight fast, giving a daily split of 12:12, 16:8, 18:6 or 20:4 (with eating hours listed second) respectively. The most popular are 16:8 and 18:6, with eating windows of eight and six hours seeming to balance effectiveness with manageability. For example, on 18:6, a person might eat only in the six hours between noon and 6 p.m. Common sense suggests eating 'normally' during the non-fasting part of the day – so you shouldn't deliberately compensate by over-overeating in your window! Eating in Ramadan is a form of time-restricted eating, where the eating window is set between sunset and sunrise (see Chapter 8).

Periodic fasting. This term is applied to choosing one or more days per week on which to fast, with usual eating (and mealtimes) on the other days – so the numbering system here is around days of the week, rather than hours of the day. One or two fasting days (6:1 and 5:2) a week are the most popular variants.

Whether fasting is a complete absence of food or an ultra-low-calorie day (some go with 500–600kcal) is more about terms and clarity rather than what you do. Having a few calories rather than a full fast may work better for some. Naturally, water and non-sweetened drinks are encouraged.

Alternate-day fasting. This is the tougher option, doing exactly what the name suggests.

Whether fasting two days per week or every other day, the idea is to find what works and feels sustainable. Time-restricted eating and fasting days can be combined – the more restriction, the more likely the benefit – so it's down to individuals to make that judgement with an eye on sustainability.

Cassie – the most health-motivated of people – used a tough combination of a very low-carbohydrate diet with two fasting days per week to maintain her T2D remission.

How does intermittent fasting work? Although its basic premise is reducing calories, the fasting windows actually do much more. Fasting helps to:

- Lower insulin and insulin resistance.

- Nurture the hormones that help us manage appetite.

- Improve the energy efficiency in our cells.

This in turn helps to:

- Reduce weight.

- Reduce blood glucose.

- Reduce the need for medication in T2D (including insulin).

Intermittent fasting is easier than daily calorie restriction for most people. If it's for you, try a month of time-restricted eating with an eight-hour food window, maybe reducing to six hours and/or adding in a 5:2 approach. Do at least a month in between adjustments, and use your sense of wellbeing, weight and hunger levels as a guide. Best not rushed.

If you are on medication, always get advice from your doctor or healthcare team – especially if you are using insulin or medication that might cause low blood glucose, such as the sulphonylurea (SU) group (see Chapter 7).

Blood pressure can fall, which is good, but be wary if you are on medication which might need reducing or stopping.

Self-monitoring of weight, blood glucose and blood pressure (Chapter 8) allows for more confident experimentation. It's probably worth tracking your sense of energy, hunger and mood before making a final judgement on its success. Adapting to an eating change is best judged over at least six to eight weeks or longer.

In summary, time-restricted eating and fasting are likely to help a lot of people with T2D, but they do involve a major change in routine.

If you are interested in intermittent fasting, the books by Dr Michael Mosley are engaging and authoritative. A medical person who has successfully reversed his own T2D, he also gives a good account of low-calorie, low-carb, and Mediterranean diets, and a number of other nutritional tips which make good sense. See Appendix 4: Further reading (for Chapter 6).

Low-carbohydrate eating

The basics were described in the previous chapter. Low-carb eating involves switching the body's main fuel from glucose (carbohydrate in food) to fat (from stores and food). In the near absence of glucose in the diet and in stores, the liver has to *make* the glucose and ketones (mini fats) to feed the brain, using stored fat to feed the body generally. Clearing liver fat reduces insulin resistance, helping restore normal function – if that's still possible. It's a neat and logical way of fuelling the body in T2D.

In all forms of diabetes, dietary carbohydrate fans the flames of raised blood glucose and liver fat, so reducing the amount in the diet makes good sense twice over.

Very low-carb eating puts us into what's called nutritional ketosis – hence the jargon term keto diet. The terminology can make it sound like a fad, which it isn't. It makes sense that it would help T2D, has been done by lots of people, is supported by lots of doctors, it works, and it has been around a very long time!

It takes two to four weeks to start to adapt to low-carb eating, during which time you may feel more fatigued (before the body has made the 'fuel switch') and light-headed – falling insulin levels allow the kidneys to excrete more sodium (salt) and blood pressure can drop. This is good, of course, but needs care if you are on blood pressure medication, and salt supplementation might be needed temporarily. Self-monitoring and working with your healthcare professional on blood pressure and medication issues are essential. A lot of people can manage their high blood pressure, without drugs, on a low-carb diet!

Research – and now momentum from practitioners – is pushing forward low-carb eating as a first-choice option in T2D. This is especially the case as people realise that food energy (calories) need not be restricted – and hunger is not usually a problem.

Longer-term, the struggle can be psychological, especially with the loss of favourite foods or the clash with the 'normal' eating of friends and family. If you are in remission of T2D, it's perfectly possible to slowly lift carb intake to see if glucose remains stable (monitoring glucose is helpful). Eating less than 50g of carbohydrate a day is a big challenge for some – and not for others. Technically, low-carb goes up to 130g/day, but above the keto level of around 50g, the possibility of losing remission is definitely higher. Again, it's that familiar ring of balancing what works for you with what you can manage long-term.

Most people have a special 'carb-miss' – bread especially. Suzanne found that remission was fairly easy with a low-carb diet and even up to the heady heights of 100g per day she kept her HbA1c in check. Her remission was maintained, and only once threatened when her wine drinking crept up. It was part of her 'ups and downs' and she addressed it. A limit of 100g per day might just allow that spaghetti bolognese dinner!

In summary, low-carb eating for T2D longer-term is very likely to be helpful. It's well researched and has endured. There would be no reason why a person achieving remission with a very low-calorie diet should not move on to a low-carb diet to help maintenance if it were to suit – the 800kcal reversal phase of low-calorie is also technically low-carb (everything is low).

Colin made the switch from low-calorie eating to low-carbohydrate eating very well after struggling with hunger on the restricted diet. He maintained low-carbohydrate eating long-term at about 100g of carb per day.

More on fat fear

Only those of us in our sixties or older can remember the time when it was normal to eat and enjoy fat. Indeed, in the generation before us – and remember people were much slimmer and rarely had T2D then – fat was revered, just as it still is in low- and middle-income countries.

Eating low-carb in T2D means eating more fat – usually a lot more than current nutritional guidelines suggest. This might bother you, or people around you. It also might bother your doctor or nurse, since guidance to limit dietary fat is still official policy around the world. If you eat a low-carb diet, and diabetes authorities *are* starting to embrace this, most of your energy *has* to come from fat. So we all now need to address this conundrum. Can we re-embrace dietary fat?

The rehabilitation of fat. The full story of how low-fat came to dominate nutritional thinking is a fascinating one – it might help some readers (see Appendix 4: Further reading (for Chapter 6) – but is optional to this section and a simple summary we feel will suffice here. First, the original scientific advice in the 1970s to lower dietary fat would not have survived current scrutiny. The connection between dietary fat and disease has substantially weakened, especially in the last ten to fifteen years.

A connection between eating fat and weight gain, although intuitive, has never been made. *Lower*-fat eating and *rising* weight have been running side by side for forty years and in practice we see the opposite. Lingering remnants of the fat–artery disease connection live on in saturated fat and its contentious link with cholesterol. Most doctors retain a belief that saturated fat is a risk to heart health, but some are now rethinking; evidence can be presented to support either view. It feels as though the jury has been sent out again to reconsider its verdict!

It is possible that a fairly small number of people would genuinely benefit from eating less fat but, for the vast majority of us, fat (saturated or otherwise) may offer no significant hazard to health – nothing like the hazard posed, for example, by T2D. If you try to reverse T2D with a low-carb diet, you will have to weigh up on the one hand a small, theoretical (or even zero) risk of artery disease from eating more fat against, on the other hand, the certainty of having T2D, which means a very real and substantial risk of artery disease. The choice might look obvious, but it's the lived experience that changes your view, not just being told by someone that eating more fat is OK.

If you opt for a low-carb diet to manage T2D long-term and/ or stay in remission, your regular blood checks and having lower blood pressure are likely to reassure you if you are still worried. If your numbers are good and you feel well, with time fat fear will disappear.

Low-fat eating, fat fear itself, some deeply ingrained habits and a highly visible carbohydrate presence in the food environment are all likely drivers of T2D everywhere.

Low-carbohydrate food options

Low-carb might seem harder if you are vegetarian or vegan, but that need not be a barrier. There are lots of food options that are good sources of protein and fat and that are low in carbo-hydrate, including mushrooms, tofu, tempeh, soy, nutritional yeast, nuts, avocados, green beans and many above-the-ground vegetables. Online help and book recipes are plentiful.

Although carbohydrate foods are nearly all metabolised to glucose by the body, they digest and raise blood glucose (and therefore insulin) to varying degrees, and of course it depends how *much* carbohydrate is actually being eaten. These features of carbohydrate foods are captured in the terms glycaemic index (GI) and glycaemic load (GL). A basic explanation and links to these terms are in Appendix 2: Terminology (for Chapter 6). In general, eating lower-GI carbohydrate foods is best.

A low-carb information and guide sheet is accessible too from Appendix 3: Resources (for Chapter 6), produced by a UK community-based medical team who managed to get half of their patients on low-carb eating into T2D remission for over two years without diabetes medication. That's a tremendous achievement.

Cutting out added sugar – but what is sugar? Well it depends whether you are a scientist, a person with diabetes, a food labeller, a shopper or none of these! There are a good few confusing terms in nutrition, but 'sugar' takes first prize by a distance.

When we eat most carbohydrates, whether simple sugars, as science calls them, or more complex starches, the body digests them directly or indirectly to glucose. Glucose is one of the body's two main fuels and the only problem occurs when we eat too much of it. We then turn surplus into fat. Glucose is a single-molecule sugar, as is the other common single-molecule sugar – fructose.

Other common sugars are double-molecule sugars. The main ones relevant to us are sucrose and lactose. Sucrose is a combination of glucose and fructose. Lactose is glucose and galactose. Galactose is a simple sugar found on its own and within lactose in milk – human, cow, indeed all animal milks. Children metabolise it differently to adults, who turn it into glucose.

So *almost* everything in the carb world gets turned into glucose – the exception being fructose. When we eat fructose, some of it gets turned to glucose in the liver, which is good. But some gets turned directly into fat – and some other unhealthy substances – which is bad. Fructose is different to other simple sugars.

Though scientists call simple carbohydrates sugars, the rest of us use the term sugar to mean the stuff we sweeten drinks or cook with – and that is sucrose.

Fructose exists in nature (mainly in fruits, honey and some vegetables) as simple fructose or as part of natural sucrose.

Sucrose = glucose + fructose

However, most of the fructose we eat comes from *manufactured* sucrose and various sugar syrups – notably high-fructose corn syrup – both of which sweeten processed foods, baked goods, sweets and sweetened drinks of all kinds. Sucrose that we add into tea and coffee, and our own food preparation, is the other main source.

Figure 6.1: Dietary sources of fructose

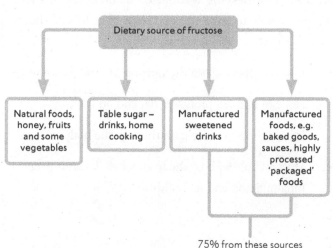

Honey is worth a mention as it's an interesting food which clearly divides people. Nutritionally, the divide is because it's a sugar syrup (mostly fructose and glucose). So is it just more added sugar to the general pool we should be looking to shrink? Or is it, as some have it, a superfood with healing properties and chemicals that enhance longevity?

Ethically, the divide is a different one, as collecting honey is considered exploitative and harmful to bees, so is off-limits to vegans. Hunter-gatherers in warm climates gather honey as a sizeable proportion of their energy intake, almost certainly with little awareness of either debate. But we are not hunter-gatherers.

The authors' summary would be to avoid honey, for both reasons. Honey is a sugar syrup and probably not different enough from other high-sugar sources to be a good choice in T2D.

Fructose provides the sweetness, naturally or unnaturally (added sugars), to our foods and most of us like it – but that's the only good bit. The rest is all bad:

• It has no specific healthy purpose that we know of.

• None of our cell processes depend on it.

• It has no easy or safe path through the body.

• Most is dealt with by the liver, where it can trigger inflammation and fat build-up.

• It adversely affects brain tissue, the chemistry controlling hunger and eating for reward, which can keep us in the 'sugar loop'.

• There is growing evidence of a link with mental health problems, including bipolar and other mood disorders, and behavioural problems such as attention deficit hyperactivity disorder (ADHD) in children.

• It increases insulin resistance, and is linked with metabolic syndrome including weight gain, T2D, high blood pressure, a raised risk of artery disease and accelerated ageing.

A controlled experiment removing dietary fructose in children with metabolic syndrome quickly reduced liver fat and improved insulin resistance just like the reversal diets do in T2D.

Glucose travels through the liver like a mature driver at the wheel of an old saloon car moving along well-established roads and carefully navigating junctions. The road, system and vehicle are in harmony; things are planned and 'regulated'.

Fructose in the liver is like a tearaway joyrider driving a sports car at breakneck speed through red lights and straight over roundabouts. Nothing is in harmony – this vehicle should not be on the road. It goes off track and way too fast. Things are most definitely unregulated. It causes a lot of damage for its small presence.

Fructose is a wolf in sheep's clothing, so why do we eat it?

Fructose has been around in food for a long time, though consumption has slowly increased. Its part-hidden presence in processed foods is compounded by confusing sugar terminology on food labels. Ironically, its metabolism and harms have only been worked out since it became a staple in manufactured foods over the last thirty to forty years.

A spoonful of sugar (sucrose) looks innocent enough, but remember half of that spoonful is fructose. Multiply that half a teaspoon by whatever you add to drinks and baking, then add in the amount put into processed and sweetened foods and drinks, and you can start to see how it mounts up.

What about the fructose in fruits and vegetables? Well, the levels are low in natural foods and their fibre 'wrapping' limits the absorption of the fructose, so eating a couple of pieces of fruit a day is probably harmless (we think!).

There's more on food labelling in the chapter resources, but if a food label says sugar or added sugars, it usually means sucrose or fructose syrup (or similar). If it's plain dairy, it means lactose (remember this double sugar does not contain fructose). It would be better to call these things by their name. Lactose, from a metabolism viewpoint, is harmless – it turns into glucose. The sugar in dairy milk is not the sugar in your pastry.

Food sugar (fructose) consumption around the world links strongly with the level of T2D. Fructose has no health benefits, so the debate in science is more about whether it causes harm and, if it does, how much and what type of harm. So there is absolutely nothing to lose from cutting out sugar and probably an awful lot to gain.

In summary, it's very likely that removing sugar (as sucrose or fructose) from the diet will help T2D, and could even reverse it.

EXERCISE

Try to work out your sugar intake

You can estimate it from food and drink labels and from what you add yourself. People use the term sugar in the food world rather sloppily – your food labels will usually say 'added sugars' or, after carbohydrates, 'of which . . . are sugars'. These terms usually mean sucrose or fructose/glucose syrups even if the names are different! Links to understanding food labels and sugar are in Appendix 2: Terminology (for Chapter 6), so if you want extra help now, go there.

The ingredients list may have one or more of the dozens of different names for sugar sources. Don't count sugar in unsweetened dairy products, e.g. plain yoghurt, milk and cream, as the sugar will be lactose (not fructose).

Look at one day, or a week if you can – use a diary or app you are familiar with. You just need a reminder of roughly how much sugar you are eating and how often you eat it.

If you can manage to get a daily figure for your sugar consumption, you have done very well. The next little challenge is to work out how that compares with recommended limits, and also to turn the figure into something you can get your head around. Five grams of sugar is roughly one teaspoon, which will do for our purposes.

The World Health Organization recommends a 25g per day limit for adults for added sugars, the UK recommends 30g per day, and many countries use 10 per cent of total daily energy (notionally estimated at 2,000kcal) which translates to 50g per day.

Adults should eat up to a maximum of 50g a day of added sugar (so not what's in fresh fruit, vegetables or dairy) which we can assume to be sucrose or an equivalent. 50g = 12 teaspoons, but various surveys suggest that typical sugar intakes in the UK, Europe (especially Germany, the Netherlands and Ireland), Australia, and parts of South America and the US exceed 70g/day and might be in excess of 100g.

The 50g/day is a guess by nutritionists. There is no guaranteed 'safe' dose of sugar, because when it comes to the fructose it contains – like tobacco or alcohol – less is better, and more is worse. So far, setting advisory limits does not appear to have had any impact on consumption.

Going back to our sample food diary earlier in the chapter (see p. 163), on two fairly innocuous looking diary days we reckon had about 60g of sugar in each day. High scorers were the sugar in tea and coffee (15g/day) and breakfast on day one, which had about 40g – muesli, jam/jelly and orange juice are common high-sugar sources. Biscuits/cookies are obvious offenders too. Main meals were relatively sugar-light.

Breakfast can be a deal-breaker with sugar. Compare porridge with cream and berries, and sugar-free coffee (almost none) to the muesli with toast/bagel and jam, orange juice and sugared coffee (40g+). Picking off high-sugar areas is not difficult to work out, but it needs commitment to put into practice.

Reduce or stop eating processed food

If you are over sixty, take a moment to think about what you remember from your childhood about life around food, how your parents shopped and ate, and how *you* ate.

Most of your meals were probably cooked from scratch using basic ingredients, which meant people were, consciously or not, controlling what they ate. Food may not have been perfect, but it was more or less real or basic fresh food.

In many countries, notably in western Europe, North America, Australia and New Zealand, pre-packaged foods make up the majority of foods eaten – up to two-thirds in some countries. The evidence linking this industrialisation of both food and the way we eat with poor health is compelling, and it's more likely than not that T2D is caught up in all of this. Eating processed foods at this level will cause sugar intakes in excess of 70g per day without people adding any to their food or drinks.

It's probably not just the sugar. High concentrations of sugar and fat together may be particularly harmful to weight and health. There are many chemical treatments in food processing which have the potential to affect health, beginning with food plant growth (pesticides) and animal rearing (antibiotics) through to the processes of mass production and chemicals that enhance flavours (different sweeteners), colours and textures, or that prolong shelf-life.

None of the chemicals used in processing foods have health benefits – it's just a question of whether they are hazardous and by how much, and whether regulation is enough to protect us all. We have to remember too that a lot of foods are processed a little – even fresh fruit and vegetables – by way of growing aids and treatments. So by processed foods we mean '**ultra-processed**' **foods** – those with a long list of ingredients which are incomprehensible to most of us and come as formulated pre-packaged meals. Ideally, eating as little ultra-processed food as possible seems best – which means eating food which has a semblance of being 'real'.

In summary, is processed food and the way we consume it likely to be worsening the picture in T2D? We think that it almost certainly is. Indeed, it's possible that eating these foods might be a major cause of the T2D pandemic.

And then there is **fibre**. It is technically an indigestible carbohydrate, and though it divides opinion, most research suggests that it benefits metabolism and can help in T2D. Its reported benefits beyond helping constipation are:

- It feeds our gut bacteria, which supports intestinal health, which in turn can benefit the immune system, reducing inflammation within the body.

- It makes for more diverse bacteria in the gut, which all the research so far suggests is good.

- It slows digestion, reduces appetite, helps with weight loss and insulin resistance, and probably reduces the risk of T2D.

- It reduces the absorption of fructose, and helps to protect the liver – which is probably why fructose in fruit impacts less than that in processed food.

Fibre supporters say we should eat 50g a day, nutritional guidance pitches in at around 30g per day, but many of us eat less than 20g per day. By contrast, hunter-gatherers have been recorded as eating up to 200g per day! If you want to increase your fibre, build it slowly over weeks and months to allow adjustment and minimise bowel discomfort such as wind!

Packaged foods tend to be low in fibre compared to foods cooked from scratch, and even if fibre is re-added, it won't nec-essarily work in the same way. Processed foods give a potential double-whammy – too much sugar and not enough fibre!

In summary, a good fibre intake probably helps health in gen-eral and is almost certain to have some benefit if you have T2D.

These are the common best food sources of fibre – there are others:

- Whole fruits (not juice) – berries are best for T2D.

- Avocado.

- Seeds – especially flax and chia (look up ways to eat these!).

- Beans and lentils.

- Leafy greens – broccoli especially.

- Nuts and nut butters.

- Whole grains.

- Oats – porridge.

- Dark chocolate – regular small amounts of the 80/90 per cent-plus cocoa stuff – yes it's bitter but does the job and you can learn to love it!

EXERCISE

Can you estimate your own daily fibre intake?

Follow labels for processed foods and look up for fresh foods. A good intake is 30–40g/day, OK is 20–30g/day and less good would be 10–15g/day or less (which is where most of us are). Estimates are OK! If you eat mainly fresh foods cooked at home, you are likely to get enough fibre.

Figure 6.2, adapted from the British Nutrition Foundation website, shows that with a bit of thought you can boost your fibre intake – in this case quadrupling it – by choosing higher fibre options with almost the same meal.

Figure 6.2: Choosing higher fibre

Fibre Boosts

Lower-fibre choice	Fibre (g)	Higher-fibre choice	Fibre (g)
Breakfast Orange juice White toast (2 slices) with jam	1.6	**Breakfast** Orange Wholemeal toast (2 slices) with peanut butter	8.3
Eat the whole fruit + 1.9g			
Snack Low-fat plain yoghurt	0	**Snack** Low-fat plain yoghurt with strawberries and almonds	5.5
		+ nuts	
Lunch White spaghetti with tomato-based sauce	3.9	**Lunch** Wholewheat spaghetti with lentil and tomato-based sauce	10.9
Choose wholegrain +4.5g		+ pulses	
Snack Cream crackers with Cheddar cheese	0.9	Snack Rye crackers with houmous	8.5
Dinner Grilled chicken breast, mashed potato and carrots	4.7	**Dinner** Grilled chicken breast, baked potato with skin, carrots and green beans	11.2
Keep the skin on +3.2g		+ more veg	
Total fibre: (% recommended intake):	**11.2g** 37%	**Total fibre:** (% recommended intake):	**44.4g** 148%

Reproduced with kind permission of the British Nutrition Foundation.

https://www.nutrition.org.uk/media/v11nc2a4/fun-way-to-fibre_nov-2021.pdf

© British Nutrition Foundation 2021 | nutrition.org.uk

The Mediterranean diet

Who would not want to eat a diet with such a name, simply oozing the promise of sunshine and health? But what is it and does it live up to that rich promise when it comes to T2D?

The Mediterranean diet is really a collection of diets inspired by traditional foods typically eaten in countries around the Mediterranean Sea, such as the south of France, Italy, Greece and the islands. They encourage the eating of fresh, real food, and are inclined towards fruits, vegetables and unrefined grains. They allow for the (largely uncontroversial) fats found in nuts, seeds and olive oil, and for poultry and seafood – especially oily fish. Dairy is moderated but allowed.

Processed meats and sugar are discouraged – in sweetened drinks, pastries, cakes and desserts, and all processed foods in general.

They get extra points for the combination of low sugar and high fibre, and are lower in saturated fat, if fat fear is still hard for you to shake! There is no reason why the basic approach cannot be angled in any number of directions to suit, while keeping to the basic principles. Omnivorous, low-carb, vegetarian, vegan or flexitarian versions are all options.

Their use correlates well with major health benefits, reducing artery disease, blood glucose, blood pressure, weight and possibly even the risk of dementia. A reduction in insulin resistance may be the reason why all these things happen. The same benefits come with low-carbohydrate, low-sugar and low-processed food (real or wholefood) diets, suggesting that the common benefit might be from reducing dietary sugar.

It's probably worth acknowledging that the Mediterranean diet, as defined and studied by researchers, may have skewed the concept of Mediterranean eating towards vegetarianism with seafood. Some feel that this plays down the many and varied meat dishes eaten in the region, but whether studied diets are traditional or not, they appear to work – especially for T2D.

People also talk about the diet being part of a Mediterranean lifestyle, which embodies at least the concept of a slower, lower-stress but active lifestyle. Eating should be slow and thoughtful, in the company of others if possible, perhaps with a small amount of alcohol. This is a somewhat fanciful and unrealistic depiction of how life and food can be for most of us – but the points remain nonetheless. Eating well – living well – for health involves *not just the food and eating.*

In summary, the research on a Mediterranean diet is robust and it's a way of eating that's been around a long time. It's likely to improve T2D and health in general, and promises to be a good long-term maintenance diet for remission of T2D. A link to an easy-to-follow explanation of the Mediterranean diet, with suggestions, is in Appendix 3: Resources (for Chapter 6).

The Mediterranean diet overlaps with a wholefoods approach to eating. The idea is to fill your plate with foods that are close to their natural unprocessed form, avoiding processed foods as much as possible. Again, it's an approach rather than a formal diet. Plant-based wholefood eating is becoming popular.

In T2D, any kind of wholefood eating is very likely to help, which in turn helps its sustainability.

Both Mediterranean/wholefood diets and fibre seem to improve our gut health – the bacteria in the intestine or 'microbiome' – which researchers believe helps with our immunity, reducing inflammation in the body and protecting us against diseases such as T2D.

Cooking

TV shows and book sales suggest a revival in cooking – though consumption of pre-cooked foods has been rising for over two decades. Perhaps we are interested in the idea of cooking but busy lives make it difficult to actually do it, and the convenience of pre-cooked food is undeniable. Which of us can say that we *always* have, or make, time to cook?

But each time we don't prepare or cook our own food, we put a little of our health into someone else's hands. The food industry ultimately targets sales – in other words wealth – not health.

Fresh basic food has everything we need for health – it always has had. The best way to eat food is to source ingredients and cook your meals; that way you can be sure nothing is missing from the natural goodness, and nothing extra – especially fructose – has been added.

Learning, re-learning or advancing your cooking skills could be the best thing you ever do for T2D. When you see your dietician, ask if there are any local courses – schools and colleges may host them. If not, ask to get one going! Maybe you have always been a good cook, but you just stopped doing it. For economy of time and money batch your cooked food, if possible, in freezer-friendly amounts. People find such simple things make all the difference.

EXERCISE

If you are more of a packet meal person, use your week-long food diary to see how many and what type of foods you've eaten, especially lunches and dinners.

Think about the reasons why you had a pre-made meal, and reflect on why you chose to do that. Examples would be: preference (favourite meal); habit; convenience; time-saving; shopping difficulty. List as many reasons from the diary why pre-made food works for you. Then list against those reasons whether you can change or challenge them, and how.

Table 6.2: Examples for food choices

Food	Reason for choice	Option to change
Chinese ready meal	Like it and easy/quick	Yes, prioritise time to cook!
Pie/veg dinner	Quick and easy	Tricky, no shop nearby for fresh veg and work long hours from home.

Vegetable lasagne	In the freezer	Frozen home-made food. No need to change.
Chips and gravy from the chip shop	Was walking past and it smelled nice	Yes, I could have a pre-pared meal ready for when I get home.
Curry, rice and naan delivered	Busy day and nothing in the fridge	Yes, I could plan my shop-ping so quick, homemade food available when I am busy.
Crisp sandwich followed by chocolate bar	Craving for something 'naughty'	Yes, avoid having foods like this in the house.

Looking at the examples above, it's clear that some forward planning and thoughtful shopping is needed to create a healthy T2D kitchen! Not having snacks and sweet junk foods in the house is going to work much better than trying to resist temptations that are on hand. What also needs to be planned for is cooking ahead for a day or two (or longer if freezing), which means a weekly food plan and a linked shopping order.

Making better food choices sometimes just comes down to making it a priority and then allocating time – and possibly (but not always) more money – to bring it about. Having T2D might mean shifting your personal goalposts in the direction of health over freedom of choice.

There are times when it can be difficult to prepare and cook food, especially if you are not the main cook in the household. Sometimes, if a person lives alone, it can feel like too much effort. If family or friends can help, great – otherwise get advice from your dietician. A little thinking out of the box (or packet) is needed. You might want to think about whether lack of time or inclination to cook can be challenged. What is your priority?

In summary, prioritising cooking could help your T2D as much as keeping active or sleeping well. If you have a friend or relative with T2D who cannot cook, help them out as much as you can – the best 'medicine' for T2D is food cooked at home.

Alcohol and T2D

An educated guess says that there are over two hundred million people with T2D around the world who regularly drink alcohol, and research on how alcohol and T2D interact is plentiful. The good news is that small amounts of alcohol are *unlikely* to pose a significant health threat in T2D, but drinking above current guidance could be hazardous. Research findings show inconsistencies, but here are the main patterns relevant to T2D:

Small amounts of alcohol – especially when taken little and often to stay within guidance – seem to carry little risk. They could even lower insulin resistance and help with T2D.

The presence of polyphenols – chemicals known to have beneficial impacts on metabolism and disease – in drinks might explain this effect. They are especially abundant in red wine, but also occur in non-alcoholic drinks and foods – dark chocolate and coffee being an appealing combination.

Drinking above current guidance and/or taking several drinks over a short time – binge drinking – increases insulin resistance and worsens T2D.

Aside from impacts on glucose and insulin, alcohol increases health risks across different diseases including cancers, and it seems the more we drink, the more likely blood pressure is to rise. If you are on insulin or sulphonylurea (SU) medication (see the next chapter), there is a risk of hypoglycaemia with alcohol.

In summary, you need to balance up *your* benefits and pleasures from alcohol with the risks. Binge, moderate or heavy drinking is bad for T2D and may shorten your life. A small glass of red wine, however, might even improve your T2D and help you to live longer. As the Swiss physician Paracelsus said, 'The dose makes the poison.'

EXERCISE

Work out your alcohol intake

The UK uses the unit (u) system for alcohol, where 1u is equivalent to a single shot of spirits, 1.5–2u to a small/medium glass of wine, and 3u is a large wine glass or a pint of stronger beer.

The recommended intake is up to 14u or less per week for men and women, spread over three days or more. Look up the alcohol guidance where you live and see where you are on the scale!

Fructose and alcohol

The metabolism of alcohol, in the liver especially, is very similar to that of fructose – alcohol is fermented sugar, and liver fat and inflammation can occur from ingesting both. These are the main shared hazards of alcohol and fructose/sugar:

- Raised blood pressure.

- Weight gain.

- Increased liver fat.

- Increased insulin resistance.

- Impairment of sleep and mental health, and a potential for addiction.

Pause for thought

Might developing T2D and/or high blood pressure make you rethink your relationship with alcohol?

In Europe and the US, up to a third of people are non-drinkers. In the UK and Australia this is only about a fifth but, interestingly, almost everywhere the number of abstainers is increasing.

There is no right or wrong here. Decisions around alcohol are personal to you.

Does it matter how we eat?

We know we shouldn't eat on the move, but we do it. We shouldn't eat while we work, but we do it. We shouldn't eat in front of the TV, food on lap, but we do it. In life there is so much to fit in, and eating is often done automatically while the 'important' things fill our headspace.

If you get T2D, it's time to appraise everything – the little things too. They may not actually be so little, and you never know what might give you an edge in health. The realisation that all is not well is hopefully enough to stop and make you think – *all* being the key word. It's not just your glucose that's not well – it's your liver, your brain, the connections and hormones of your body and more. It's the way you think and the way you live.

Ted was not the only person to be surprised by the diagnosis of T2D, most people are. It's understandable, even when we are retired and less busy with big things, that headspace can fill up with things 'outside', and we are not used to giving time to consciously thinking about the mechanics of looking after ourselves. We take sleeping and eating for granted, but all the signs are that we shouldn't.

Can we complement better food choices with a better eating style – one that helps health? Well, people think so, and plenty of research suggests that more thoughtful, slower eating can help not just with digestion, which we've always accepted, but by helping us to eat less and, maybe, with weight control.

Is the benefit of the Mediterranean diet about the food or the ambience and experience of eating? If we eat quickly because we have no time or are too busy – or it's just a bad habit – we deprive ourselves of the physical benefits that quality eating can bring, and the psychological and human benefits too.

Research suggests a direct link between slower eating, less weight gain and a lower risk of T2D. Eating a meal for thirty minutes or more allows a fullness sensation to develop in time to prevent overeating. If thirty minutes sounds long, try at least twenty!

EXERCISE

Use a timer to see how long it takes you to eat your main meals

How far are you off twenty minutes? Now try slowing down and using a twenty-minute alarm! We will flag this up again in Chapter 8 when we look at being a self-manager. You might be able to see if being more thoughtful about eating has had an effect on how long you spend sitting at dinner, and in turn whether this is reflected in the results of any monitoring that you do.

Eating thoughtfully

Have you ever been driving and arrived at a point with no strong memory of the last couple of traffic lights or junctions? Have you ever caught yourself eating while watching TV and just looked down and found your plate was empty, with no memory of having actually swallowed your food? Sometimes, lost in thought, we go into full-on automatic pilot.

It's obviously more dangerous driving a car than eating a TV dinner – but the latter is not without hazard. Switching off when we eat, whether whilst watching TV or scrolling/looking at a screen, means we easily miss the cue of fullness and can overeat. On a single occasion, it's no problem, but done regularly over a long period it could impact our weight.

This is the opposite of mindful eating, which helps us to be aware of all the sensations of eating, which in turn help us to sense body cues better. People have found that they can become intuitive eaters – knowing when hunger is hunger and not boredom, and when to stop eating. Thoughtful eating means not clock-watching, and allowing time for body signals to develop during a meal. After finishing your plate, you can tell if the body needs a little more food after twenty minutes, not twenty seconds!

If you live alone, it can feel harder to focus on eating well, but try not to eat with TV, radio or screen distractions; try relaxing music instead, and use that twenty-minute pause after eating before thinking of extra food or dessert. Conversely, if you live alone, you may find it easier as you only need to be concerned about your own eating. When living with others it can be challenging to stray from the rest of the household's eating habits, with greater temptation and pressure to eat in a certain way. Either way, there are challenges and it is important to acknowledge them.

You can read about mindful eating, following the link in Appendix 3: Resources (for Chapter 6).

Eating processed food quickly is the most unhealthy way to eat, on multiple levels. Eating real food more slowly and thoughtfully is healthy on every level. If your way of eating is a cause for concern, and you have T2D, try to get help; the same applies if you are struggling with retaining remission or have been advised that you are at risk of T2D. A nutritionist/

dietician might be able to help you rethink your relationship with food and offer strategies for dealing with the negative impacts on your health and staying positive.

Eating tips from the experts – those people successfully managing T2D

These are a handful of things that many people with T2D have found helpful in managing their own eating:

- **Eat in the same way every day if you can** – not the same food, obviously, but as with sleep, try to develop a good routine around mealtimes. Allocate enough time to enjoy and eat thoughtfully.

- **Drink water** – though tea and coffee are OK (watch the caffeine). Water flavoured with fruit and different varieties of tea can add some variation.

- **Don't snack** – not buying snacks in the first place can help you do this.

- **Don't buy what's not on your food plan** – emptier cupboards are good.

- **Celebrate your achievements**, such as improving your weight or HbA1c. Celebrating what you have done, rather than not done, helps you to stay positive.

- **Self-monitoring can be powerful** – giving feedback to help you understand how what you do affects your body. Tracking blood glucose (if possible), blood pressure, weight, exercise, eating and hunger can all keep you in charge of your health (see Chapter 8).

Addressing food storage to deal with casual overeating is probably one of the most effective single ways to stay healthy. If, on the odd occasion, hunger gets the better of you, reflect that we are all human and try a handful of nuts – most are very T2D-friendly. **How you shop is an integral part of managing T2D**.

So what can we summarise from this whistlestop tour of long-term eating and T2D? Well, *something* has to explain what's happened with T2D! It's likely that more than one thing is at work, but underlying are still the simplest of questions. If we are overeating, *why* are we? Are we eating too much carbohydrate? If so, is it too much of all of them, or just the simple sugars? Drilling further down, might fructose – present in everything that's bad and low or absent in everything that's good – be the 'lone gunman'? Eating little or no processed food would be a simple if challenging approach to long-term eating for health, and very likely to work.

Given that we need a better strategy than the one we have, as individuals let's encourage each other to think openly and not be bound by the blinkers of a single approach. One approach is almost certainly not going to work for all people with T2D.

Our suggestions:

If, after reading this book, you retain your belief in the importance of calories, then try some form of intermittent fasting rather than cutting back every day. It's more likely to help.

If you think that lowering carbohydrates might be worth trying, then why not start by getting rid of as much sugar as you can from your diet – a no-risk strategy if ever there was one!

Eating little or no highly processed food gets rid of most of the sugar problem and helps with fibre. Cooking more is partly about regaining control. The food industry is not part of the health industry but maybe it should be.

The Mediterranean diet could be the least contentious of all diets available for T2D, and it is accessible to all. It can be tweaked towards T2D by adjusting carbohydrate downwards (more vegetables from above the soil-line, less from below) and allowing for vegetarian, vegan or flexitarian versions.

If we ate this way (the food *and* the way of eating), we are convinced that T2D itself could start to go into reverse.

This and the previous chapter have been about food, but using FAST at every step can remind you that other things are important too, and that things are very much joined up.

Key points from Chapter 6

- We should start to think about healthy eating as what individuals do to stay healthy, free of disease, with good energy, stable weight and a healthy liver.

- Diets are theories or models, not absolute facts, and should be viewed more open-mindedly.

- A successful long-term eating plan needs motivation and commitment to sustain it.

- Feeling better is a powerful motivator.

- Standard nutritional advice is not always helpful for managing or preventing T2D.

- Low-carbohydrate (or low-sugar) eating, intermittent fasting and the Mediterranean diet (or similar wholefood diet) are all likely to help T2D long-term.

- Eating fewer (ideally no) processed foods would be good.

- A quality eating experience – slower and more thoughtful – helps metabolism and T2D.

- Shopping and food storage are key parts of successful eating plans and reducing snacking.

- Eating healthily is full of options – if you've been diagnosed with T2D, the only one not to try is the 'more of the same' option.

Type 2 diabetes and staying safe

T2D and risk

If T2D was just about the symptoms of raised blood glucose, its treatment would simply be a matter of using one or other of the drugs that lower glucose. Symptoms would then either improve or go away. Unfortunately, this is not the case. T2D can cause artery disease, whether blood glucose is controlled or not; medics nowadays think of T2D itself as an artery disease. This chapter is mainly about trying to keep your arteries healthy.

Disease of very small arteries – such as those in the retina of the eye, around the nerves under the skin and in kidney tissue – can damage eyesight, and can cause loss of feeling and kidney failure. The higher the blood glucose, the more this type of damage impacts. Though it occurs in both T1 and T2 diabetes, it's more typical of T1D.

The second type of artery disease affects larger blood vessels – those taking blood around the body to larger organs such as the heart, the brain and the limbs. Disease of these blood vessels can lead to heart attacks, stroke and poor leg circulation (amputation if severe). This pattern is more typical of T2D. It is not uncommon to get both types of artery disease in T2D.

Do these patterns tell us something? The small blood vessels are particularly susceptible to injury from the glucose level itself. Although it's the very 'stuff of life' at normal levels, when it's too high, glucose damages the blood vessel lining. So small blood vessel damage connects with higher blood glucose levels in any form of diabetes.

The larger blood vessels are damaged by a different mechanism – maybe more than one – and this includes insulin resistance, which is why T2D also causes this different pattern of artery disease. Insulin resistance – which connects with strokes and heart attacks – occurs in people without T2D, though, as we are learning, the diabetes can be rumbling along in the background or might appear later. Insulin resistance also links with high blood pressure and both contribute to this pattern of artery disease.

Improving your blood glucose will reduce your risks from one type of artery disease (microvascular or small vessel disease) and improving your insulin resistance will reduce the risk of the other type (macrovascular or large vessel disease).

Colin suffered a heart attack and was diagnosed in hospital as also having T2D and high blood pressure. Insulin resistance will have been the driver for all three. Treating his blood glucose will not improve his insulin resistance, so while his risk for small artery disease will improve, his risk of further heart attacks remains. Lowering his blood pressure will most definitely help to lower his risk of a further heart attack.

The United Kingdom Prospective Diabetes Study (UKPDS) 1977–1997 has guided thinking on the medical treatment of T2D around the world. Its main lessons, which continue to inform, have been that:

- Lowering blood glucose reduces the damage to small arteries in T2D – so less eye, nerve and kidney disease.

- Lowering blood glucose has much less effect on damage to larger arteries, so less impact on heart attacks and strokes.

- The oral diabetes drug metformin *does* reduce large artery disease.

- Lowering blood pressure is at least as helpful as lowering blood glucose in preventing both types of artery disease.

- Most people need four or five medications to manage blood glucose and blood pressure.

- Acting earlier in the disease improves your chance of *staying* healthier.

The UKPDS meant that medical treatments of blood glucose and blood pressure intensified, possibly at the expense of a focus on diet, which is the main way to lower weight and insulin resistance. It also showed us that blood pressure is just as, if not more, important than blood glucose in preventing harm.

Most people with T2D have high blood pressure because insulin/insulin resistance raise blood pressure – they go together.

Insulin resistance is the best predictor of serious long-term health problems in T2D.

Intensifying medical treatment gives a reduction of about a third in the risks of artery disease – maybe more or less on an individual basis. But getting that level of benefit from medications is not always straightforward, since pills can have side-effects, and insulin has the added risk of hypoglycaemia (low blood glucose). In the medication world, benefits always have to be balanced with harms.

Macrovascular disease

Before we go further, we need to look at large blood vessel artery disease just a little more, as it is the major complication of T2D and medication for glucose has only a modest effect. This type of artery disease is the commonest cause of death in people all over the world.

T2D is one of the major links to, or causes of, artery disease – along with long-term mental illness or stress, and smoking. High blood pressure can either be viewed as a separate cause of artery disease or a link with T2D through insulin resistance. It depends on how you look at it.

It's worth reflecting on this for a moment, because a major aim in treating T2D is to prevent artery disease, so it makes sense to join up a view of T2D with other known causes of artery disease. If you have a significant mental health problem of *any* kind then that needs to be managed as well as possible to reduce its *physical* impacts – which can include causing or worsening T2D and artery disease. Managing stress and strain has as much impact on your physical health as on your mental health. So if you have T2D, prioritise managing your mental health as much as your blood glucose – they interlink. Remember FAST.

Neither stopping smoking nor managing stress and mental illness is easy but try to shine your light on more than one thing and it might just pay you back. Treating depression in T2D is indirectly also treating the diabetes and potential artery disease, which is why Colin so typifies the challenge of T2D; there are more twists in his journey . . .

T2D and a different kind of 'heart' disease – when sex goes AWOL

Well before his diagnosis of T2D (and his heart attack), Colin had become significantly depressed, with work-related stress and money worries. He was so low that managing his T2D was difficult, and antidepressant medication made little difference. His blood glucose improved a little on his diabetes medication. A few months after his diagnosis, he was referred to a psychological therapist.

In the year before his diagnosis, he had been experiencing erectile dysfunction. His relationship with his wife was good, but the problem of sex was undiscussed and unresolved. His self-confidence was very poor. He restarted smoking as a stress-reliever – a habit from years before which he realised later just made things worse. His heart attack happened in a swirl of physical and emotional issues.

Problems with sex are common in life, especially as we age, and are more common again in T2D. We know that diabetes causes erection problems for men, because the blood vessels and nerves of the penis are not working well. But while this is better understood in T1D, the mechanism in T2D seems less obvious – ageing and psychological issues may also be involved.

Women with T2D experience sexual problems too, but there is sadly much less research and understanding. Sex and happiness are inextricably bound; we know that regular sex makes us less stressed and healthier. Research tells us that T2D causes sexual problems, but we don't know if helping sexual problems can help with T2D. It might.

Colin's depression slowly improved in therapy, and more so when he was made redundant. Losing his job had been his main worry, but it turned out to be on more favourable terms than he had imagined. With lifting mood came a returning interest in sex. His erection difficulty improved with sildenafil (a drug for improving erection) – but even more so when his therapist talked with Colin and his wife as a couple.

Two years after his heart attack, Colin was still on diabetes medication with a HbA1c of 52mmol/mol (7.1%). He was much happier; things were working better and he had read about T2D reversal.

Sexual problems in T2D are common, and many of us feel uncomfortable talking about them, but, if improved, it can make for a better life and can maybe help T2D too. Like reversal, you can't know if you don't try. Colin's problem could have been from artery disease or psychological stress – or both. What matters is that both can be improved. Colin was lucky to have a therapist who asked the right questions.

Many people avoid discussing sexual difficulties, which is a pity as solving such problems can be as life-changing as achieving good glucose control (things which might well connect!).

Artery disease

The source of T2D and artery disease is wrapped up in insulin resistance; treating that is largely about changing what and how you eat. Managing that along with improving fitness, sleep and tackling stress might feel like a big challenge. But the effort involved is less than treating established T2D or living with the consequences of artery damage. Prevention is not just better than cure – it's easier than cure. Things well known to prevent or lessen artery disease are:

- Put T2D into remission, or significantly improve it, lowering blood glucose and blood pressure.

- Manage or prevent stress/low mood and improve mental health.

- Stop smoking – definitely don't start!

- Take a statin (explained shortly).

There are a few less well-known things too and we'll mention those later in the chapter.

Hyperglycaemia – raised blood glucose – is the main target of medical treatment. As we've explained, medicating it downwards can only prevent a proportion of its risks, but it's still worth doing well. For context, normal blood glucose (and related values for HbA1c) are shown in the table below.

Table 7.1: How HbA1c and blood glucose connect in T2D

HbA1c		Equates to	Average blood glucose	
mmol/mol	%		mmol/L	mg/dL
42	6.0	Below 42 (6.0) is normal	7.0	126
48	6.5	42–48 (6.0–6.5) is borderline or 'at risk' of T2D	7.7	139
60	7.6	50–60 (6.7–7.6) T2D is 'OK'	9.8	176
70	8.6	60–70 (7.6–8.6) scope for action	11.0	198
80	9.5	80+ is over 9.5% treatment usually maximised (including insulin)	12.5	225

Ideally, for good control, you will want HbA1c to be as close as possible to normal or the diagnosis threshold of 48 (6.5%).

Decision points and review

The first decision point is when you are diagnosed – whether that be with T2D or as being at risk of T2D.

Two of our case examples – Ted and Cassie, aged seventy-eight and fifty-six respectively – showed how different the decisions can be after a diagnosis of T2D. Ted had a HbA1c of 56 (7.3%) at diagnosis, relatively low, with only minor symptoms, and felt well overall. He had opted not to try to reverse his T2D (Chapter 5), instead choosing to follow standard dietary advice and to do more walking. After a slight improvement in weight and HbA1c, the trial was extended but, after a few more months, no further progress was made and Ted agreed to try metformin (coming up shortly).

Cassie's HbA1c was over 100 (11.3%), and she was advised by her local specialist team to use insulin, at least as a temporary measure. But she struggled with the thought of this, and having read up on the possibility of reversal, opted to try dietary reversal. As we saw in Chapter 5, this worked well for her. She agreed to use metformin too, but then had to stop because she developed diarrhoea – a common side-effect. With a safety net of glucose self-monitoring, and easy access to her nurse and doctor by phone, she was able to watch her glucose steadily drop during the early weeks. Although a confident and assert-ive person, Cassie could not have managed this easily or safely without support. Discussions with her diabetes nurse, mainly on the telephone, were weekly initially.

First treatment decisions can normally be reviewed at two or three months, on the basis that other things are happening too – you should have early access to diabetes healthcare education and a full baseline physical assessment. With time, the decision or review points can be every six months or so. The key thing is that they are purposeful, and while orientated around an agreed blood glucose (HbA1c) control target, they should give time to assess diet, activity (exercise), mental wellbeing and sleep – in other words, how you are living. Every discussion is an opportunity to think beyond glucose. A review point after a change of medication will need to allow up to three months for a HbA1c test to show the impact of the change.

Keep your review active and thoughtful. If nothing has changed between review points, still try to use the opportunity to think about all of your T2D, not just medication and glucose numbers. Raise any questions that you have and use a quick mental FAST check to cover all the ground relevant to T2D:

* Am I happy with the plan – is medication to target HbA1c on track?

* Am I doing what I can to help my T2D? Think about eating, weight, being active, sleeping well. Do I need help or advice with any of these important areas?

* Am I in a good place mentally – does anything need sharing?

A shared and accessible plan is a must, however it's generated – paper printout, computer summary, copying on to your tablet or phone. Its contents should include the things that identify you, a summary of your background, health history and current medications, what has helped and what hasn't, and your up-to-date T2D plan. You can refer to it anytime, carry it with you if you travel or go into hospital for whatever reason.

Medications to lower blood glucose

We are not going to list all the drugs that can be used, but a simple summary of the main ones might be useful. We are using only proper (scientific) names for drugs, not the manufacturers' names – both will be visible on packaging.

Metformin is the most important drug in managing your glucose in T2D. It's not quite one of a kind, but it does more than just lower blood glucose; it almost 'nudges' metabolism in the way that the right food can. Discovered a hundred years ago, it was found to lower blood glucose quite by chance. It works in the liver and in the gut and hormone systems of the body, and the latest research suggests that it works inside cells to improve how we handle energy; all of which give clues as to why it protects against artery disease.

Metformin is continuing to reveal its benefits decades after it came into use. It's not a superhero drug, but it comes close, and if you can tolerate it, take it! Metformin's one downside, however, is its tendency to irritate the gut by causing nausea, sickness or diarrhoea. It's not serious, but is irritatingly common, affecting up to one in four people. Building the dose slowly, or trying different versions of the drug, occasionally helps. Being so beneficial, it's worth persevering, but sometimes the side-effects can be just too much. If you are one of the lucky ones who are OK with it, it gives a good first base, and some people can manage their blood glucose on metformin alone, even for a few years.

Ted felt well on metformin only, and had a small drop in his HbA1c to 50 (6.7%). He had the benefits of a slightly lower glucose and additional artery protection from metformin. It's a balanced way of looking at things and, importantly, Ted was happy with it. He was relaxed in his life, which is good for his metabolic health!

If you need medication but are intolerant of metformin, then there are other options, in three main groups (there are others depending on what's available to you). Older drugs, other than metformin, are still in use:

Sulphonylureas are sometimes shortened to 'SUs'. If you take a tablet for T2D ending in -ide it will be an SU. Common examples are gliclazide, glipizide and tolbutamide. They work by stimulating failing pancreas cells to just keep going and make as much insulin as they can. This *potential* benefit can also explain their common side-effect of weight gain and their main risk of hypoglycaemia. A blood glucose reading low enough to cause symptoms – hypoglycaemia is usually below 3.5mmol/L (63mg/dL) – is not common with tablets, but can be difficult to treat. Metformin and an 'SU' was always a popular combination, but SU use is likely to decline as medicines gradually improve.

'Flozins' and 'gliptins' are the main newer start-up drugs. The flozins are so called because all the drug names end with that, for example canagliflozin (they are all equally difficult to pronounce). Similarly, gliptins all end with those letters, for example sitagliptin (they are marginally easier to pronounce!).

Flozins work by causing the kidney to excrete more glucose (so there's less in the blood). They are well tolerated but extra glucose in the urine can trigger infections just as it does when T2D starts up! Flozins (as with metformin) offer a little extra protection against artery disease, so are used for people who are at extra risk. Colin, for example, was treated with metformin and a 'flozin' because of his heart attack.

Gliptins work to help stimulate insulin and slow down digestion, helping fullness when eating. They also reduce glucose manufacture in the liver and, though their impact is not massive, they are easy to live with.

Injectable medications which are not insulin are starting to be used more. This group are the 'GLP-1s' and they help the body to produce more insulin if it's needed, and to reduce the amount of glucose the liver makes when it's not needed. They can help with appetite and may help weight loss. Examples are exenatide, liraglutide and dulaglutide (there are others – all ending in -ide). There is a medication guide table, including the newer injectables, in Appendix 3: Resources (for Chapter 7).

In summary, metformin is the first choice of medication, if tolerated. The older drugs (SU group) are tried and tested but can cause weight gain and carry a risk of hypoglycaemia. Newer drugs, such as flozins, are easier to take and, along with metformin, offer a little protection against artery disease, as well as lowering blood glucose. All drugs have pros and cons, and none is perfect.

It's common to move from one drug (usually metformin) to two in the quest to reach your target HbA1c. Under 48 (6.5%) takes you out of the diabetic range; under 53 (7%) is excellent; up to 58 (7.5%) is still quite good, and fine for many people. Beyond that is a judgement that you have to make – balancing the wish to get HbA1c as low as possible against having to take more medicines and risk an occasional side-effect.

Decisions on adding medication, especially insulin, can be complex and need to consider your age, personal circumstances, other health problems and medications – as well as your own choice! Wise choices come from shared decision-making with your healthcare team. A link to an example of a treatment decision aid in T2D is in Appendix 3: Resources (for Chapter 7). It is from the UK's National Institute for Health and Care Excellence (NICE). You may find it useful, or something similar may be accessible to you locally.

Each interval review gives you an opportunity to check your status against your agreed target HbA1c and, equally importantly, to reflect on that target and see if it is still right for you. Over a number of years, most people will end up on maximum therapy which might be three drugs, but the journey to that point will vary between individuals. Insulin resistance and gradual loss of insulin secretion varies between people in an unpredictable way, and blood glucose might stop getting worse, if only in spells, if diet and exercise push things in the opposite direction.

Without remission, especially if T2D comes on before the age of fifty to fifty-five years, you are likely to need insulin to manage glucose/HbA1c at some point. Only a very low intake of carbohydrate, minimising the need for insulin, can delay or partly control that. Eventually, T2D can become like T1D in respect of insulin – it goes missing!

Insulin is often recommended if you are running out of oral medication options, or if you have troublesome diabetes symptoms and poor control – internationally reckoned to be a HbA1c of over 75 (9.0%), in spite of maximum efforts in medication and lifestyle. The first step in practice would be to consider the impact of insulin – injections and effects – for you as an individual.

Pause for thought

What might injections and using insulin mean to you?

If you are in your fifties, and T2D is your only problem, using insulin is a more straightforward proposition than for someone in their eighties, with multiple problems, medications and restricted mobility, who perhaps lives alone. For those unable to make their own decisions, a judgement will fall to professional and family carers. Sometimes the decision is not whether to use insulin, it's how – how easy will it be? How many injections a day? And who will give them?

Insulin treatment always involves more than one person. Family, friends and colleagues need awareness, occasionally training, and ideally access to written information and 'what-to-do' guidance.

Injection worries

Using insulin feels serious and some anxiety is natural. However, in reality, unlike with T1D, there is time to adjust, prepare and practise.

For 95 per cent of people, self-injecting quickly becomes second nature. Most of us have mild needle phobia, but after a few try-outs with needles that are so fine that a scratch is an exaggeration of their impact, it passes. If you have a major needle phobia, you may find the self-help book *How to Beat Fears and Phobias* by Mark Papworth helpful – see Appendix 4: Further reading (for Chapter 7). Psychological therapy can also help – sometimes it can be as little as one session – and everyone really gets there in the end.

Insulin can be started whilst still taking metformin. The main things to know about the different insulin preparations are:

- How long they work for – a few hours (short), many hours (intermediate), or up to and over a day (long).

- How long they take to *start* working, and when their peak action occurs in the bloodstream.

- How many injections are needed to suit your circumstances.

- How to store and manage 'the gear'.

- How to self-inject (or give injections if you are a relative or carer).

- How to manage a 'hypo'.

- Who (and how) to contact for urgent advice.

- Last but not least, insulin causes weight gain – just like too much natural insulin does.

Using insulin is mainly about knowing its action – the time it takes to work, when its effect is peaking and how long it lasts in the system. Knowing these things for the insulin you are using is all you need to know about the theory. In practice, *you* have to work out how insulin works in *your* body, with *your* activities, foods and moods! This means monitoring. Self-monitoring of blood glucose is covered in the next chapter.

Many people with T2D have been routinely treated with long-acting insulin injected once a day, usually at night. Twice daily preparations are a mix of short- and long-acting insulins (two in one). The short-acting component helps to manage the glucose arriving in the next meal, and the longer-acting component helps to manage the glucose in the following meal and beyond. Injections are given before meals. The short-acting insulin component may have a peak action in the bloodstream at two or three hours, whereas blood glucose from a meal peaks at one or two hours or so – rather earlier. There needs to be a gap between injecting and eating therefore, or the two things may not connect well. Managing this gap between injection and food is something to be learned.

Mustafa uses a twice daily insulin mix, and injects before breakfast and dinner or main meal. He adjusts the timing of his injection to take account of his mealtime, and to some extent what he is eating. He has used self-monitoring of blood glucose to learn how his body reacts to different foods and the injection/food interval.

It's mainly the carbohydrate in the food which causes the glucose to rise after digestion, so eating meals which are mainly fat needs much less insulin. Glucose control and insulin issues (and doses) are inevitably less on a low-carbohydrate diet. Even with T1D, there are now many people – including doctors who have the condition – who are finding life easier and possibly safer when carbohydrates are restricted.

Insulins given once a day (often called background or basal insulins) in T2D have no real peak and connecting them with mealtimes and other activities is unimportant. If you are new to insulin, learn the basics about the insulin you are on and learn from monitoring yourself. Your healthcare team will help, but the real experts on insulin are those who have managed it long-term for themselves – more in Chapter 8.

Hypoglycaemia ('hypo') is a blood glucose below 3.5mmol/L, however you may not be aware or able to check your reading. Your healthcare practitioner will have provided you with written instructions on what to do but, more importantly, those instructions should be available to your family (and friends if need be).

If mild, the symptoms are like anxiety – feeling shaky, sweaty or hungry. More severe symptoms can be difficult to manage if they involve confusion, as others may see an agitated or irritable person and be unaware of what's happening. It can be really difficult to manage if a person has been drinking alcohol, as this can provoke a hypo, and an onlooker wouldn't know whether slurring and confusion was the alcohol or low blood glucose – carrying an alert device that says you are on insulin could save your life.

Most hypos involve people using insulin and are avoidable – missed meals and unplanned exercise are common triggers. However, you might not be aware that hypos can occur with oral medications too – especially the older SUs we mentioned earlier, where low blood glucose can persist for much longer and be unresponsive to oral glucose. Hospitalisation is sometimes needed. If you take an SU, you have to be aware, so self-monitoring of glucose is strongly recommended. Metformin does not cause hypos.

You will not be started on insulin without full education and written guidance around avoiding and managing hypos – but be aware that those close to you need to know what to do and where your hypo kit is kept!

Using insulin can be a problem if you drive a car or operate machinery in your work, and you might be faced with a difficult decision. You may be allowed to work with blood glucose testing as a safeguard. Your healthcare practitioner will support the transition to insulin and will be familiar with driving regulations.

Managing hypertension (raised blood pressure)

High blood pressure is important – it has risk implications, and can be a marker for insulin resistance – which is why it is so strongly linked to T2D and why managing it is *just* as important as managing glucose.

Measuring blood pressure is best done at home, and allows you to get familiar with the numbers and the way that it varies with time of day, recent food, and especially exercise and tension levels. Follow the guidance from your healthcare team, use a reliable recommended machine, and remember to record the result if the monitor does not have built-in memory.

These are the blood pressure numbers and action points:

- Normal: less than 135/85.

- Level 1 elevation: 135/85–149/94 (over 150/90 if aged 80+). Take action, medication may be required.

- Level 2 elevation: 150/95 or more. Take action, medication is probably required.

- If on medication for raised blood pressure, the target is less than 135/85 (or 145/85 aged 80+).

This guide is based on self (home) monitoring of blood pressure, and ideally on multiple readings, taking an average rather than a single reading. More on this in Chapter 8.

Home monitoring helps you stay in control and connect with what's going on – it may even help to lower your blood pressure. It's also a convenient way to check the impact, favourable or otherwise, of a change – whether it be medication, a dietary alteration or a change in life circumstances. In all these situations, judge your blood pressure over a two-, three- or four-week period.

What can make your blood pressure high?

- Insulin resistance.

- Sleep problems.

- Medications for arthritis (see later).

And too much:

- Dietary salt.

- Alcohol.

- Caffeine.

- Stress.

If T2D can be reversed, blood pressure nearly always drops, and medication can be stopped. A low-carbohydrate diet, even without much weight loss or T2D reversal, may still improve your blood pressure, as can drinking less alcohol, being more active and improving sleep. If you are stressed or anxious, and can manage its cause, do so. Relaxation methods can be as effective as blood pressure medication. FAST applies to blood pressure just as it does to blood glucose.

If self-help is not enough to keep blood pressure within the guidelines, medication will be needed. High blood pressure impacts the arteries in a person with T2D at least as much as raised blood glucose or smoking. This makes blood pressure targets lower and multiple medications are more often needed. Self-help is complementary to medication in blood pressure control and can reduce the number of drugs and the risk of unwanted effects overall.

T2D and statins

Statins are recommended for most people with T2D, to help reduce the risk of artery disease. They were introduced more than thirty years ago to help reduce cholesterol, which at that time was thought to be the main risk factor for artery disease. Individual drug names all end in '–statin' (simvastatin, atorvastatin, etc.). Their value and use provoke debate, even within the medical community. This is a debate which is really beyond the scope of our book, but be aware that:

- Statins lower cholesterol overall, but that *on its own* is no longer thought to be relevant to artery disease.

- They help to protect the blood vessel lining – which is how some experts believe that they work (i.e. not to do with cholesterol at all).

- They have been associated with causing muscle aches, fatigue and a potential risk of *causing* T2D – somewhat concerning if you actually have the disease or are at risk of developing it.

- Medics who are sceptical about statin use still believe that they work – that is, they lower risk – but the risk reduction is quite small, making their overall value much less clear-cut than you might think.

Is it really worth taking a statin? No definite answer is possible and we accept that most people will follow the guidance of their own doctor in this controversial area. If you would like to read a thoughtful analysis of the subject, check the blog by Professor John Worrall (link in Appendix 4: Further reading (for Chapter 7)).

The impact of reversing T2D or stopping smoking would be far more than any potential benefit from a statin, which in any event you could discard if you were in remission – unless you are convinced by those that say everyone should take one!

T2D and smoking

Smoking is linked with T2D and the liaison is a particularly dangerous one. One in four or five adults around the world are thought to smoke, though thankfully the overall rate is slowly declining. The proportion of people with T2D who smoke is probably a little higher, and smoking is regarded by some authorities as an independent risk factor for actually causing T2D.

T2D and smoking each more than double the risk of artery disease, including heart attacks, stroke and limb amputations. For a person with T2D who smokes, the risks are much higher. Stopping smoking is one of the biggest health-improving changes you can make – *especially if you have T2D*.

Most smokers say they want to quit and have tried at least once. Simply stopping on your own, with no strategy except teeth-gritting, succeeds in only about one in fifteen or twenty attempts. You can increase that chance significantly by getting help, such as taking part in a smoking cessation programme, which often uses medication to help with the addiction part. A lot of people relapse, but the success rate long-term can be improved modestly and is worth a try, given the big benefits.

You can appeal to any number of sensible thoughts with smoking and other similar addictions, but they tend not to help; saving money has been studied, and motivates a few folk, but without some deeper motivation, the habit pulls you back. You could ask what greater motivation there could be than having a diagnosis of T2D, and knowing that you are doubling an already high risk to life and limb by smoking. But sometimes we don't process risk well, and especially if our mental health is not good.

Colin admitted after his heart attack that he had been secretly smoking over the previous year. An ex-smoker, he had quietly slipped back into his old habit when work-related stress took over his life. It didn't work, he admitted later, and probably contributed to his heart attack – maybe even his T2D.

There is no magic bullet to stop smoking. Health shocks sometimes work, but that's not ideal! Colin was lucky, in a way, that his heart attack did not affect his heart's performance, but managing risk for him had urgency – though that was difficult for him to see through a veil of depression.

We think that a psychological approach to quitting smoking is more likely to help a person quit long-term than the assisted teeth-gritting of medication and nicotine replacement. With smoking, we sometimes build ourselves up to fail by making it feel harder to quit than it really is. An approach that encourages some repositioning of thoughts around smoking, minimising the scale of the addiction and the difficulty of quitting, will be more successful. After just a few weeks, any physical addiction is gone. Memory and habit linger, but you are on your way.

If you think you could never enjoy going out socially without having a cigarette, then remember that the large majority of people now don't smoke (including many ex-smokers) and they are happily enjoying their social lives, and so can you.

Links to help with smoking are in Appendix 3: Resources (for Chapter 7) and in Appendix 4: Further reading (for Chapter 7). Find more information to make quitting more likely to happen.

Pause for thought

Key inner motivation is unique to you. The risks from T2D with smoking are as high as health risks go – what do you value most in life?

There's more to artery disease than 'just' T2D – say yes to NO (nitric oxide)

The lining of our blood vessels can be prone to inflammation, clots forming on the surface and blockage of the vessel itself – which we all hope to avoid. T2D, smoking and stress are big causes and high blood pressure is a strong connected risk factor, but is there anything else we can do to try to keep our blood vessels healthy?

Here are three suggestions to help lower your risk of artery disease which don't involve taking more medication – one involves taking less! They make scientific sense, have stood the test of time and have extra health benefits too. The following tips all involve promoting the level of **nitric oxide**, a compound of nitrogen and oxygen, commonly known as NO, which helps lower blood pressure and improves blood vessel (lining) health. It's an incredibly important natural substance around arteries, and we know that its level can be reduced in T2D. (Note that nitric oxide is not related to nitrous oxide, or laughing gas, which is an anaesthetic somewhat hazardously used recreationally by some people to produce a high.)

1. Relaxation – putting aside short periods in your day to relax, meditate, take deep breaths and be mindful can reduce blood pressure, strains on the body and risk to the heart and circulation as much, or more so, than any medication. This is endorsed by medical specialist organisations. We covered aspects of relaxation in Chapter 4. Combining spells of relaxation with deep breathing through your nose brings even more benefit by boosting levels of NO made in the inner lining of the nose. That's extra benefit from NOse breathing! (See Appendix 3: Resources for Chapter 7.)

2. Sunlight and fresh air – nitric oxide is also stimulated in the skin by exposure to sunlight, on a 'the more the better' basis. This can lower blood pressure and promote healthier blood vessels. Combining exposure to sunlight with exercise can lift mood on both counts, and improve your vitamin D level if that's needed. So as part of your FAST approach, consider putting fifteen minutes a day aside to relax with deep breathing (remember the NOse) and a daily walk in fresh air and sunlight.

3. Reducing medication risks – as we get older, medicines can be more difficult for the body to handle and side-effects become more common. Non-steroidal anti-inflammatory drugs (NSAIDs) – the ibuprofen/naproxen family – are in common use for age-related osteoarthritis and many other, mainly rheumatic, conditions. NSAIDs can irritate the stomach lining and are often given with stomach-protecting drugs called PPIs (the omeprazole/lansoprazole family). Osteoarthritis and T2D occur in roughly the same age group, commonly people aged over sixty.

As it happens, both NSAIDs and the PPIs that are used with them increase the risk of artery disease by adversely impacting the blood vessel lining and reducing nitric oxide manufacture. They can also unintentionally increase your blood pressure.

NSAIDs are not life-savers and their effectiveness often wears off with regular use. This small but definite increase in the risk of artery disease and blood pressure might matter if you have T2D, and could make you rethink their use. NSAIDs are widely used (probably overused) worldwide. Glucosamine may be worth considering as a long-term and safer alternative to NSAIDs if you have T2D or related metabolic disease and intrusive symptoms from osteoarthritis. It's been used for a long time and has a low-level effect on inflammation in joints and, more generally, on associated pain. Accumulating research evidence suggests that the benefit might be more than we thought a few decades ago, and it appears to be very safe. It's being mentioned here because of the observation that glucosamine users seem to experience some protection from artery disease – and if you have T2D this might matter. T2D and NSAID treatment is not the best combination; T2D and glucosamine might be a safer and risk-reducing combination. Note: glucosamine sounds like glucose but it's not really related. It is connected to some of the structures that we see in joint cartilage. A review article explaining a little more about glucosamine is in Appendix 3: Resources (for Chapter 7).

If you have T2D or are at risk of T2D and are taking one of these medicines, try to establish whether it's helping you. Stopping it for two or three weeks is usually enough time (you can always restart) or ask your doctor or pharmacist to review your medications. Every little helps with T2D and risk.

Key points from Chapter 7

- Managing raised blood glucose lowers some of the risk of artery disease.

- Improving insulin resistance by diet and weight loss will reduce that risk by more.

- Controlling blood pressure is as important as controlling blood glucose.

- Metformin is the first-choice medication in T2D.

- Insulin may be unavoidable in late T2D, but insulin management is easier and safer if lower doses are used, which means a lower-carbohydrate diet.

- Preventing artery disease in T2D can involve different approaches, not typically connected with the T2D itself.

- Reducing or avoiding smoking is as important as controlling blood glucose and blood pressure.

- Keeping arteries healthy is the main aim of treating T2D, and self-help is the key to both.

Type 2 diabetes and being in control: be a self-manager

If you have T2D, you are likely to see your healthcare team for less than two hours a year. The other 364 days and twenty-two hours you manage yourself! Being a good self-manager can be critical to the outcome of your T2D. Most good outcomes are said to be delivered by people themselves, not by their health-care team. In other words, delivered by *you*.

In Chapter 7, we looked at the usual medical management of T2D, which is focused on managing both blood glucose and blood pressure, and the measures that can be taken to help you keep your arteries healthy. Doing these things along with your own self-caring requires a treatment plan, some monitoring and a well-coordinated effort between you and your healthcare team.

In this chapter, we're going to explore why being a good self-manager can help you to stay in control, reduce your risk *and* help you to stay well. Self-managing in T2D is partly based on self-monitoring, which means knowing what you are doing – understanding how to interpret things, and ideally how to make helpful adjustments to what you are doing.

T2D presents a special case for self-monitoring because it is a disease of the way we all live, so looking at the way *you* live is the beginning of being responsible for getting yourself back on track.

Monitoring and review of T2D

Traditionally, these have been coordinated and carried out by healthcare teams using a framework developed by doctors. Increasing use of insulin in T2D has meant more self-monitoring of blood glucose, and more people now monitor their own blood pressure.

Renewed interest in dietary treatment of T2D means more dietary monitoring – much of which can be done, with suitable support, by you. Self-monitoring can be done on most things that can impact on T2D and health, such as sleep. So monitoring is a mixture of things done by your healthcare team and things that you do for yourself.

Review. A literal meaning of review is to look again, and what we do, either in healthcare teams or for ourselves, is to look again – often at key measurements such as HbA1c – to track its journey. The review incorporates elements of monitoring into a framework, and we use it to answer two main questions:

1. How are things going compared to before? Are they better? Worse? Steady?

2. How are things against our aims or targets – such as, am I sleeping better? Am I following an agreed exercise plan?

Review then concludes with a judgement about whether change is needed. Do we need to adjust something? And is the target – for example for blood pressure or HbA1c – still appropriate?

Healthcare team monitoring. This is done at intervals, and is usually clinic-based. Its main elements are: interval tests such as HbA1c, and checks of liver and kidney function; examinations such as those to check the circulation and nerves in your legs and feet, and the retina at the back of each eye; validating and cross-checking any self-monitoring information, such as home blood pressure, weight or foot checks; and dealing with current issues or problems, such as any new symptoms.

Colin didn't mention his erectile dysfunction in clinic, but it was uncovered later by his psychological therapist. Margaret had a spell on metformin during which time she had mild diarrhoea. A change of the tablet formulation settled the problem.

Healthcare team monitoring should always be able to cover the necessary checks, deal with issues and carry out a review of where things are. The process should also allow for a reflection on key support areas, following FAST or your own/team version of something similar.

Successful healthcare team review hinges on a good medical record – preferably shared – whether written or electronic, and your own personal record-keeping/diaries. This also allows for better interactions with people who are not familiar to you – such as staff changes and problems when you are away from home.

The healthcare team review is often about balancing 'the numbers' and covering *your* issues and problems, and its frequency is dictated by circumstances – Cassie was reviewed weekly early on when she was unwell. When things are stable this might be every few months or even once a year.

Annual review. Damage to arteries is what underlies the so-called complications of T2D, though we now think of them as part of the 'vascular burden' of the disease. An annual review is designed to pick up and address early signs of artery disease – both the small arteries which supply the tissues of the kidneys, eyes and nerves of the body, and the large arteries which carry blood around the body.

Kidneys and eyes are checked because kidney failure and sight loss are a big part of what can go wrong in T2D. Kidney tests are lab tests and you would have no way of knowing if your kidney function was declining until it was well advanced. If your healthcare team pick up a problem, they will want to make sure your blood pressure and blood glucose (HbA1c) are as good as they can be, and will advise you about medication doses and what drugs to avoid.

Checking your eyes is essential to detect any blood vessel damage caused by T2D, which can be treated directly (on the back of the eye) to prevent sight loss. Tell someone if your sight changes – it might be that you need new glasses or a cataract checked (usually an easy fix) or it could be that your blood glucose is raised or changing, and it is that which needs attention rather than your eye.

Disease of the retina is serious in sight terms, but much can be done to protect and save vision. An annual check of your eyes is one of the most important things that you can have, but at any point, tell someone (your healthcare practitioner, optometrist/optician or eye specialist) if your vision changes.

Although these are technical areas of diabetes care, and you don't carry the checks out yourself, you do have a big role to play in both as: **both kidney and eye problems can be prevented and helped by focusing on blood pressure and blood glucose and by improving your T2D overall.**

As with eyes and kidneys, foot checks are, in part, checking the health of the smaller arteries by making sure that the nerves in your feet are working properly. By checking the pulses in your legs and feet they also give an opportunity to check the health of larger arteries. Being able to check the health of both small and large arteries makes the foot check just about the most important part of your physical examination.

Foot checks are also a little different because they come more into your direct control – they can be part of self-monitoring. For example, you might have had a very recent foot examination and then develop a problem which needs prompt attention. T2D can make you more prone to infection and inflammation – a poor healer if you like – and you might leave something longer than you should before getting help, especially if a recent clinic check was reassuring.

Some leg and foot problems come from glucose damaging the small blood vessels that nourish the nerves under the skin.

Reduced sensation means you might not feel how hot your bath is or that you've stood on something sharp; skin easily gets damaged, inflamed or infected. Ageing circulation is usually neither perfect nor terrible – most of us are somewhere in between. Wherever you are on that scale, in T2D, damage to the skin of the legs and especially the feet can trigger a vicious circle of inflammation and possible infection. It's important to nip things in the bud – and to do that you have to be vigilant. Don't ignore anything new, whether your last check-up was a year ago or a week ago.

Ted had been to an educational talk on foot care. It was not long after this that he noticed a small red mark on the side of one ankle. He couldn't remember a rub or injury, but he knew to mention it. His healthcare practitioner checked his feet generally, which were OK, but he had a small skin ulcer, which took a month to heal with treatment.

Some skin ulcers in T2D take months or longer to heal and occasionally break down again. By being vigilant, Ted prevented a much worse problem. **A really good habit is to have a close look at your feet once a week**.

- Sit and look at your bare ankles and feet, check the soles, and if you can't see them, use a mirror or get someone else to look.

- Anything new to see?

- If you see any redness, small cuts, blisters or sores, can you explain them?

- Is anything rubbing? Have you noticed any change of shape in your feet or toes?

If you feel or see anything you can't explain or something doesn't look right, speak soon to your healthcare practitioner. Foot problems can make life a misery. A foot check can be done once a year by a healthcare practitioner, but can also be done every week by *you* – both are important. It's simple. If you don't already do this, please start.

Ask for written information on foot care or find it online. Podiatrists or foot doctors will see you as a priority. Always wear comfortable shoes or trainers with support insoles and try to avoid walking in bare feet.

Muscle pains when you walk can be a sign that larger blood vessels in the leg are becoming narrowed. There are no medications for circulation problems, but tell your healthcare team, as you will need closer supervision. Disease of other large arteries (those involved in heart attacks and strokes) are not assessed directly, but they are part of the same circuit as the leg arteries, and they are protected best by good control of glucose and blood pressure, taking a statin and not smoking. Managing your T2D as best you can ties in well with what your healthcare team is doing. Self-care and medical care work best together. It's obvious why self-care makes all the difference: healthcare teams are mainly *checking* things, while you are mainly *doing* things!

Monitoring weight, whether in clinic or at home, is often so routine that only its connection with the last reading is held in mind – is it up or down? Is it stable? But now that we know that T2D can be reversed by the loss of internal fat, and that a total weight loss of around 15kg (33lb) helps to achieve this, a target weight of 15kg below that at diagnosis might also be held in mind. If you are lean or have a normal BMI, that weight loss target could be 10kg (22lb) or even less.

If rapid reversal of T2D has not been attempted or sought, it's still probably worth keeping that weight target; getting close to it by slower weight loss could substantially improve the T2D at some future point. If your weight is stuck, think about what you've read in Chapters 5 and 6 – there are options.

Self-monitoring

T2D without any self-monitoring is like being a passenger in a car with a driver whose mind is on other things. You can see vaguely where you are going but really have little say in the route taken, or even the destination. Being a passenger of your T2D is OK if you really don't want to drive. But choosing to drive 'under supervision' and then driving a little more on your own means you have some control over your own journey.

Self-monitoring by definition is part of self-help, and though it has always been there around tracking blood glucose if you are on insulin, this should now also include weight and blood pressure. We are making a case here to think about self-monitoring of anything that might impact on your T2D – small gains can add up to big differences. These would be self-monitoring of:

- Blood glucose even if not on insulin.

- Blood pressure.

- Food and eating.

- Weight.

- Exercise.

- Sleep.

- Low mood or stress (anxiety).

Self-monitoring and self-management are like learning to drive – the effort takes time, but that gets less as things become second nature. Eventually you don't need to ask, 'How am I driving?' – you just *are*.

Some years ago, John knew someone with T2D named Jean, a lovely older lady who made being in control of her T2D an art form. She spent a set time each day on her diabetes journal, looking at her blood glucose readings, her food and mealtimes, when and where she walked, and how her spirits (mood) were. She was on insulin but had good glucose readings and rarely got even near a hypo. She observed the way her eating, activities and insulin connected up. Jean monitored her blood glucose, insulin dose, blood pressure, weight, exercise and mood. In Jean's time, we didn't realise how important sleep was – or she would have monitored that too! Her commitment to being in control helped make her life as good as it could be. Somewhere in Jean's approach is the key to living well with T2D.

Self-monitoring connects you with T2D – if you want that. Psychologists tell us that self-monitoring raises awareness of – and curiosity in – our condition. It makes us more accountable for how we behave in relation to our health, and fosters a kind of self-competition – we *want* to do better. Doing better means we keep a better check on the things that we can with T2D. It also makes us ask more questions, or look things up. We become better problem-solvers. But self-monitoring is not for everyone.

We are not all enthusiasts, though comments from researchers suggest that this can stem from a lack of explanation or support from healthcare teams. We need to know what self-monitoring is for and feel that it makes a difference.

Like most changes, we see the same three key components:

- To be a successful self-manager you need to know how and why monitoring something can help (knowledge).

- You have to be willing to try monitoring to see whether and how it helps you (what works).

- The inner belief that it's all worthwhile (motivation).

These elements interact and sustain each other.

Benjamin had been self-monitoring his blood pressure for years, and was able to adjust the dose of his medication, within reason and with clear written guidance from his healthcare practitioner. As a result, his blood pressure control was very good, which helped both him and his healthcare practitioner have confidence in that part of his care. But it also made him much more aware of how his medications worked and why blood pressure was important to manage. It made him read more about this and about other aspects of T2D. Overall, he felt more engaged in his own care.

If you are newly or recently diagnosed – or even if not – you should be able to access a formal in-person or online education programme. In the UK, there is DESMOND (Diabetes Education and Self-Management for Ongoing and Newly Diagnosed), which is open to all people with T2D or those at risk. Most countries seem to have a version of this, and if not, you should be able to access what you need directly through your health-care team. This is a minimum. Try to take every opportunity to learn about T2D. Check the explanations, resources and suggested reading for relevance to you, on T2D subject areas, in our Appendices 2, 3 and 4. There are also a number of links to online presentations – from what is HbA1c, to gathering your motivation to tackle T2D. People who self-monitor often say how much that makes them want to find out more. There are books in our suggested reading, Appendix 4, on exercise, sleep problems, low-carbohydrate eating, intermittent fasting, reversing T2D, living with insulin, depression, problem-solving, metabolism and stopping smoking. We have learned so much from reading, and so might you.

Charities, non-profit organisations and healthcare organisations everywhere can offer help and support through chat, talks and meetings online and in person. If you are not confident online, ask your healthcare team for guidance. Experts by experience are the real gems of diabetes education.

Ted's wife had a friend with T2D who introduced him to a local group – people with T2D and partners or carers who met every month in their village hall. Guests might do a short talk on something relevant to T2D, but of course the main event was socialising and exchanging T2D stories!

Ted learned a lot about foot care from a visiting podiatrist (for which he had cause to be grateful as we saw earlier), which persuaded him to look at his own feet much more closely and more often.

Knowledge around specific monitoring

If you monitor anything, you learn – no matter your knowledge before you start. This is because it's not theory anymore, it's what's actually happening for you. We have emphasised for a reason the importance of food, exercise, sleep and mental health, as some part of one or more of these things will be driving your T2D. It is for you to judge which factor(s) and how.

Reflecting on this with people close to you and your healthcare practitioner might help with your focus. It's helpful to have an idea as to why T2D might have happened – think back or re-read the first four chapters if need be.

You can monitor everything without outside help, but it's better to share the experience with your healthcare team. Because wider self-monitoring is not normally covered in a standard interval review, this is a learning curve for everyone.

Back to Benjamin. When he made adjustments to his medication, they were always communicated to his healthcare team, who updated his main medical record so that his prescriptions and any blood tests were always made clear. We can call Benjamin a self-manager, but he worked in tandem with his team.

If you are new to T2D, or have not thought too much about it and would like to make a start on understanding your own T2D, try using a diary for two or three weeks, or longer if you can. Talk this through with your healthcare team and plan a meeting or some way of sharing the information.

See Figure 8.1, a suggested page-a-day diary example for T2D lifestyle. It has space for recording food and drink, activity/exercise, sleep, mood, tension, recording blood pressure/blood glucose/weight and space for reminders and comments. Use or adapt the blank version in Appendix 3: Resources (for Chapter 8). Your healthcare team may be able to help. There is no perfect monitoring diary out there; most are for T1D and used mainly for tracking blood glucose. Ours acknowledges FAST but you could design your own!

A lifestyle diary is not meant to be too detailed or complicated but to give an overall picture of, for example, the type of foods you eat, how much you exercise and sleep, and how you rate your mood. More detailed work might be needed on an individual area. When we diary something we get a better idea of what we do rather than the vaguer notion of what we *think* we are doing. When tackling T2D, knowing what you are *doing* is as important as what your tests show.

This would capture most of the information lending itself to self-monitoring but not in the detail that, for example, a sleep diary would give about sleep on its own. Think about the sections on the diary page, but if you prefer you could make up your own version to suit. Tracking your 'bigger picture' for, say, two to four weeks, could help you and your healthcare practitioner see which areas you might want to address. Blood glucose can be recorded here if you are on insulin, and/or have access to self-monitoring – *and* find it useful.

Don't worry about getting things right or wrong, this is not a research tool, or for other people – it's just for you to understand your own patterns. If your diary identifies sleep as a potential problem area, then do a more detailed sleep diary, looking at the duration and sleep quality (see Chapter 4).

Monitoring can go further. We suggest you track your sleep against food, alcohol, exercise and mood, again for maybe two weeks. You might spot patterns: 'I sleep longer when I don't eat after 7 p.m.' 'Drinking any fluid after 9 p.m. nearly always makes me get up to pee in the night.' 'I seem to sleep longer when I've exercised early that day.' Or 'I sleep better/worse/longer/shorter after alcohol.' All are possible – but remember alcohol sleep is not the same as healthy sleep.

Don't forget to track your duration of eating at some point – especially that of your main meal. Longer eating times help fullness to develop properly and limit overeating. Have you become more thoughtful about spending longer over meals since reading Chapter 6? The aim was to eat your main meal

Figure 8.1: Example diary page for daily monitoring of T2D

Page a Day: Self-Monitoring Diary for T2D

Date: 13.06.2023

Breakfast	Blood Glucose	Activity/Exercise
Oat Porridge Berries Yoghurt Black Coffee	Before: Time: After: Time:	Before breakfast: Brisk walk for 45 mins 5 p.m.: Exercise bike for 30 mins

Lunch	Blood Glucose	Sleep
Mushroom Omelette Orange Mint Tea	Before: Time: After: Time:	Number of Hours: 8.5 Sleep Quality: (1 = Poor, 5 = Excellent) 1 2 3 (4) 5

Tea/Dinner	Blood Glucose	Mood/Tension
Pan Fried Fish & Sauce Steamed Veg Crackers, Butter & Cheese	Before: Time: After: Time:	Mood: (1 = Very low, 5 = Good/Happy) 1 2 3 (4) 5 Tension: (1 = Calm/Relaxed, 5 = Very Stressed) (1) 2 3 4 5

Symptoms, Issues and Problems

Tender side of right big toenail but nothing to see – keep an eye.

Drinks and Snacks

Nuts 3.30 p.m.
Mint Tea
Water with each meal

Measurements

Blood pressure: 134/82
Time: 10 p.m.
Weight: 82.3kg

Reminders for the Day

Try to check BP at bedtime
Eye check next week

over at least twenty minutes or so. If you change something – say, the time of your last meal – you can diary the next two weeks to see if there is benefit. You can experiment with this kind of diary approach, balancing value against effort. If you value sleep more than the time you eat your dinner, then you can make a helpful change, e.g. eat earlier.

Use the information from Chapters 3 and 4 on sleep and exercise to think about whether you need to do anything at all with these things. If you exercise regularly and sleep more than seven hours at night, these are not your priority areas.

If low mood or stress is a persistent problem, bear in mind that it will affect T2D, perhaps more than you think (see Chapters 10 and 11). Don't play it down and, at the very least, ask your healthcare team about extra help. If mood is intermittently a problem, can you see any patterns from your diary? It might be worth doing one for a whole month in that case. Low mood can connect with poor sleep or having blood glucose readings out of range (only detectable if you self-monitor), and commonly it can link with alcohol use.

For most people, a more detailed food diary is the thing that you might need to master. If you or your healthcare team feel that you need to change your diet for T2D, it would help to have a diary and support from your team. The dietary options we listed in Chapters 5 and 6 are not all mainstream yet in T2D, but neither are they unheard of. Your healthcare team will probably guide or supply you with information, or else check Appendices 3 and 4 – that's Resources and Further reading – for Chapters 5 and 6.

For a major diet change, especially to the increasingly popular low-carbohydrate option, you should see a dietician with a background in T2D – preferably one familiar with low-carb eating.

Monitoring blood pressure and blood glucose are valid and easy ways of assessing if/how changes in food, exercise, sleep and stress management are working for you – which really can help you improve both.

Figure 8.2: Monitoring – what and why?

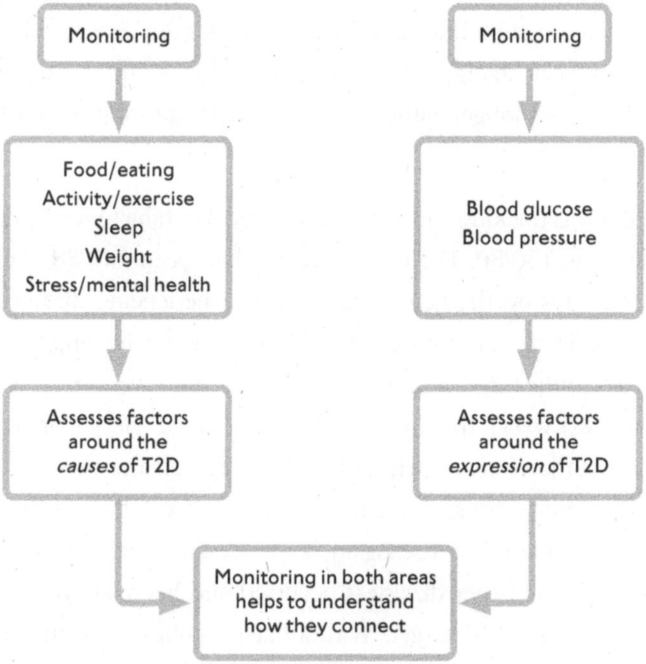

```
┌──────────────┐                    ┌──────────────┐
│  Monitoring  │                    │  Monitoring  │
└──────┬───────┘                    └──────┬───────┘
       ↓                                   ↓
┌──────────────────┐              ┌──────────────────┐
│   Food/eating    │              │                  │
│ Activity/exercise│              │  Blood glucose   │
│      Sleep       │              │  Blood pressure  │
│      Weight      │              │                  │
│Stress/mental health│            │                  │
└────────┬─────────┘              └────────┬─────────┘
         ↓                                 ↓
┌──────────────────┐              ┌──────────────────┐
│ Assesses factors │              │ Assesses factors │
│   around the     │              │   around the     │
│  causes of T2D   │              │ expression of T2D│
└────────┬─────────┘              └────────┬─────────┘
         │        ┌──────────────────────┐ │
         └───────→│ Monitoring in both areas │←─────┘
                  │  helps to understand     │
                  │   how they connect       │
                  └──────────────────────┘
```

Self-monitoring of blood pressure

Monitoring your own blood pressure is the most straightforward of things if you take time to learn to do it properly and use a reliable and recommended machine (check with your healthcare team). If you're new to this, arrange a review after a few weeks to look at readings, check your technique and deal with any queries.

Monitoring blood pressure is especially helpful after starting or changing related medication, or adjustments in diet or alcohol intake, but is essential when attempting reversal of T2D or switching to a low-carbohydrate diet for any reason. Blood pressure can change within days but might take up to a month or more, so longer rather than shorter monitoring would be best.

Colin was tracking a medication change. His target blood pressure was 130/80. His recent average had been 142/88. After a few days on the new drug, he was experiencing dizziness, especially on standing up. His blood pressure readings were closer to the target and his dizziness was not severe. However, after two weeks there was no further change. He telephoned his healthcare team, who advised a week off the new medication and to try again. The dizziness stopped, but his blood pressure started to rise again, so he restarted medication as agreed. No further dizziness occurred and his readings stabilised closer to the target. Without self-monitoring, Colin and his healthcare team would have struggled using only clinic readings; self-monitoring of anything is generally more useful than clinic monitoring on its own.

Self-monitoring of both glucose and blood pressure has taught us that 'good' clinic readings of both can hide significant swings which have meaning.

Suzanne's home readings showed that borderline blood pressure dropped when she stopped drinking alcohol for a few weeks, and also that her night-time readings were low or normal but much higher in the daytime. Suzanne struggled for some time with this balance but the knowledge that alcohol impacted her blood pressure stayed with her and helped motivate her later to moderate her drinking.

Having daytime readings much higher than those at night can be a sign that stress is a factor and using alcohol to relieve stress is not straightforward.

Checking blood pressure at intervals of three, six or even twelve months is less likely to pick up changes that might need attention than does more frequent self-monitoring. Of course, it's about getting a balance. Check frequently when needed, perhaps daily for two or three weeks when diagnosing raised blood pressure, monitoring medication or other changes (especially diet), and then at longer intervals when things are settled – the detail is up to you with the advice of your health-care team.

Self-monitoring of blood glucose

Everyone has HbA1c checked with T2D, but not everyone self-monitors blood glucose. HbA1c is a really reliable test, and has become the standard for diagnosis and decision-making in general. However, as with blood pressure, this 'interval' measurement reflecting average blood glucose can hide meaningful variations.

Blood glucose is raised in T2D, but it can also be more variable (larger up and down swings) within a given day or between days. Though better understood in T1D, research suggests that these excursions of glucose matter in T2D too. They are associated with a higher risk of artery disease and also hypoglycaemia, which is highly relevant if you are on SU medication or insulin (Chapter 7). Monitoring blood glucose would allow a person to detect and link variations in readings to treatment, food and exercise in particular; adjustments in one or more of these might help to smooth out glucose swings to a more normal pattern.

Jean was doing this without formally understanding the harmful impact of the variations themselves. She intuitively thought that it was a good idea to keep things steady – and she was right!

Figure 8.3: Blood glucose variability

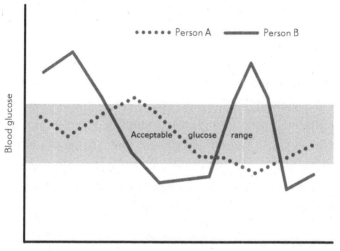

Here we see the blood glucose readings on a particular day of person A and person B, who we have imagined to illustrate this particular point, and that their readings on other days were similar. A and B have the same HbA1c but B's blood glucose readings show much more variation, both high and low. Having readings within or close to the grey band is best. A's readings are more stable, which is better for health.

When HbA1c isn't useful on its own

Self-monitoring of blood glucose can also be useful when a HbA1c reading is unexpectedly high or low. Let's say a person's reading went up from 55 (7.2%), which is good, to 76 (9.1%), which needs attention. An occasional fasting/morning glucose reading was only a little above normal, but later in the day, after-meal readings were much higher than usual. More detailed monitoring using a food diary might then help that person to get back in control.

Other than finding the answers to questions like 'Why has my HbA1c gone up?', self-monitoring can also be used to quickly collect information on glucose control. If a person changed their diet on 1 January, HbA1c will show the impact of that from mid-March onwards (assuming the diet is continued). With glucose self-monitoring before and after the change, the effect can be seen over one or two weeks.

Cassie used glucose self-monitoring to help with her food choices on the low-carb diet which had taken her into remission. She also used a regular early-morning blood glucose reading to help her monitor her T2D overall. It gave her confidence knowing that things were steady.

Cassie was using her new knowledge of T2D alongside a high level of motivation to avoid losing her remission, and overseeing what worked for her body in terms of food and glucose. These three things again – knowledge, motivation and 'what works for you' – are powerful and self-reinforcing.

The value and motivation for self-monitoring of blood glucose is personal, and deciding whether to do it has to be tied in with availability and costs. Guidance on how to perform glucose self-monitoring is in Appendix 3: Resources (for Chapter 8); and on its place and value in Appendix 4: Further reading (for Chapter 8).

Self-monitoring expectations and problems

It can be really helpful to match expectations from monitoring to knowledge of the area that's being monitored. Weight is the best example of where we can all underestimate the timescale of change. Unless a very vigorous dietary change is employed, weight needs to be judged over months, not days and weeks. HbA1c changes are also gauged over a similar timescale. Changes in blood pressure and glucose can be reliably interpreted over a shorter timescale – days to a few weeks.

There is also potential to see change more quickly earlier in the course of T2D. We know it's easier to prevent or reverse T2D early on rather than when the disease is more advanced. The body's systems have more scope for the change. Monitoring the impact of sleep, exercise or diet changes on T2D of twenty years' duration may be less and/or slower than when the disease has just surfaced.

But just occasionally, expectations need to be lifted and the best example is probably weight again. Whereas when we change the way we eat, we have to give adequate time for it to work, we don't need to go for too long either before we judge it *not* to be working. Progress within two or three months should be seen – definitely by six months. If you go that long with no progress you are standing still and need to rethink your plan – especially around food and eating. We should have low or no expectations that being stuck is OK. It isn't.

There is no real downside to self-monitoring so long as it's done with an understanding of its purpose, is supported by healthcare teams and is valued by and helpful to the person doing it. We see this particularly in the area of glucose monitoring where Cassie's experience shows how remarkably effective it can be when done by a motivated and well-supported person.

Research on self-monitoring – including that of blood glucose – is yet to explore its potentially rich possibilities; healthcare teams and people with T2D need to make this journey together to realise those possibilities. If you feel anxious about self-monitoring it may be that explanation and support is all that you need – its role, techniques and tactics should be part of your healthcare team review. But ultimately it's your T2D and your decision on whether self-monitoring is for you.

We can see just how important monitoring can be when the body is not in its usual rhythm, such as during illness or when we fast for whatever reason. Of course, there is overlap in the body of these two states.

Fasting with T2D – Ramadan

For Muslims, Ramadan is a time of heightened spirituality and sense of community, and involves adults and older children fasting in the hours between sunrise and sunset for thirty days each year. There are well over a hundred million Muslims with T2D. Every year, they experience the spiritual uplift as well as the practical challenges of managing T2D during daylight fasting.

Ramadan poses extra challenges for those on insulin, during hot weather and when the daily fast is prolonged. At high latitudes, the summer solstice can mean an eating window during darkness as short as five or six hours a day.

We met Mustafa in Chapter 1 and looked at the impact of shift work on his health in Chapter 4. Originally from Iraq and now living in the UK, he developed T2D in his early fifties and is currently treated with insulin and metformin. He made a trip to his home country to visit family, his first since he developed T2D and his first Ramadan on insulin. His GP, also a Muslim, helped with the trip planning, giving food and drink guidance, a checklist of things to take, including medications and a hypo plan. Mustafa also did some pre-travel practice fasting!

In Ramadan, his fasts were around twelve hours long. He was using both insulin and metformin tablets twice daily. He continued metformin but took a larger proportion of his daily insulin dose in the evening and a smaller dose in the morning.

The challenges of Ramadan with T2D are those of blood glucose variation (high and low) and dehydration, especially in a hot country. Advice is generally to medicate for night as day and vice versa, in line with the reversal of eating patterns. Eating should be pitched to avoid too high a blood glucose overnight and early morning, and too low a reading during the daylight fast. Food energy should be apportioned fairly evenly across the two meals at Iftar (evening meal) and Suhoor (morning meal), with the latter taken as late as possible before daylight. Sugary foods and drinks should be avoided.

Exercise should not be strenuous during the fast and, from a T2D viewpoint, evening prayers should be regarded as exercise. Self-monitoring of blood glucose more often than usual is the key to staying safe, especially if you are on insulin or hypo-prone oral medications, and drinking lots of water is important.

On one day, Mustafa felt sweaty and dizzy in the late afternoon. He had been walking and assumed it was the heat. He rested and checked his blood glucose, which was low for him at 4mmol/L (72mg/dL). He was reluctant to break his fast, so he rested for longer and rechecked his glucose but it was still fairly low and, faced with a long wait until dusk, he safely and sensibly took oral glucose to prevent a further drop in BG. After this, he limited his exertions in the afternoon period and experienced no further incidents.

Not fasting is an option within Islamic guidance, as is breaking a fast to avoid a health risk as Mustafa did. Most people with T2D are not at high risk during Ramadan and sensible precautions and flexibility are all that's needed. There are some excellent sources of information on T2D and Ramadan, covering all aspects, including suggested food adjustments. See the links in Appendix 3: Resources (for Chapter 8).

Ramadan should be a great experience, and one that can enhance health. Fasting can be good for T2D – limiting consumption is fundamentally not going to harm you, especially if you are on no medication. A well formulated low-carbohydrate diet is perfect for Ramadan, but changing the way you eat just before or during Ramadan is definitely *not* a good idea!

If you smoke, for all the obvious reasons Ramadan could be a good time to stop.

Illness and T2D

It can be worrying when you have T2D and experience any form of illness, commonly an infection, especially one that interferes with eating, and more so if you are on medication. Frequent questions include, 'Do I still take my tablets?', 'Can I take other things?' and 'Do I need to get medical help?'

Surprisingly, expert guidance differs from country to country, and even within areas of the same country. We've pulled together here the advice and practical points which are, in the main, agreed.

Firstly, if you have T2D you should know what to do if you get sick, and this especially applies to illnesses which include vomiting or diarrhoea, and where appetite has gone or eating and drinking are difficult.

An illness plan should be written and accessible to you and your family or carer and should be reviewed at least annually with your healthcare practitioner. It should be personal to you, based around your experience, how your T2D is managed and whether self-monitoring of blood glucose is accessible to you. The plan should show clear instructions on when and how to access professional help.

Have a sickness pack containing things that help minor illness and hypoglycaemia, and a glucose self-monitoring kit if available. Here are some practical points to keep in mind:

- Blood glucose usually rises during illness, even when you are not eating – remember most of your glucose comes from your liver, not from your food.

- If you are on insulin, don't stop it – you may need more – so use your written guide to manage that, as it will vary according to the type of insulin you use.

- Take extra fluid on board – water only is best. Two to three litres per day, sipping 100–200ml or so every hour if you can manage.

- Eat as you normally do, if you can. If appetite has gone, either sip easy-to-digest soups and drinks or stick with water, which is fine for two to three days.

- Monitor if you can – blood glucose in the range 5–15mmol/L is safe. If it's not stable, check several times each day.

- The problems of illness come more often than not from dehydration, so if you feel dry (thirsty, dry mouth, headache, lethargy) take more care and get advice; your healthcare team will welcome that.

- If on oral medication, continue it if you can, but if you are vomiting or think you might be dehydrated, get medical advice on any medication you are taking, whether for T2D or high blood pressure. If medical advice is not available or is delayed, stopping oral medication is usually safer pending guidance.

A link to an example of 'sick day' guidance is in Appendix 3: Resources (for Chapter 8).

Benjamin picked up a bug one day. His wife had shaken it off a few days before. He had vomited for a couple of days, with mild diarrhoea. On day three, he was struggling to keep water down and felt unusually lethargic, with a bad headache and dizziness. He wondered if his blood pressure might be high. He self-monitored so checked the reading which, to his surprise, was unusually low. His pulse rate was high.

His wife called for advice. The doctor knew Benjamin and his medical background and, suspecting dehydration, arranged to visit him at home. While waiting for the doctor, Benjamin tried to stand up, fainted and badly cut his head. Worried, his wife phoned for an ambulance.

Benjamin had low blood pressure and a rapid pulse because he was dehydrated. His blood glucose was near normal but tests of his kidney function were not. His diabetes medications were stopped and he was given an intravenous drip (fluids IV) and felt much better within forty-eight hours.

This was a one-off episode for Benjamin. The infection that made him vomit was not serious, but the dehydration and his diabetes medication combined to stress his kidneys, making him much more poorly than a simple bug would have.

Self-monitoring of blood pressure triggered the original call for advice.

Self-monitoring, whether it be the impact of food on weight, sleep on glucose or illness on blood pressure, is a way of staying in control, having the means to help you improve – or sometimes just keeping safe.

Key points from Chapter 8

- Healthcare team monitoring is professionally led and should be shared with you. Self-monitoring is led by you and should be shared with your team.

- Self-managing is being able to monitor and make adjustments to improve your T2D.

- Always mention problems to your healthcare team.

- Checking your own feet regularly is a good habit to have.

- Keep in mind a target weight of 10–15kg below your weight when you were diagnosed.

- Anything that impacts T2D can be monitored and the information used to try and make helpful changes.

- Self-monitoring of blood glucose is essential when using insulin but useful in other situations.

- Minor illness in T2D is much like minor illness without

T2D, but always follow written sick day rules; continue insulin but get advice on oral medication.

- Monitoring blood pressure is easy and is mostly something to do at home.

Suzanne's story: diabetes, pregnancy and the metabolic boom

Diabetes in pregnancy is either something you already have going into pregnancy or it occurs only in the pregnancy, disappearing again after you deliver your baby – this is called gestational diabetes mellitus or GDM. Historically, T1D has been the main type of diabetes going into pregnancy. T2D used to be very uncommon in women of childbearing age but is now more common than T1D in younger women. GDM, also uncommon in the past, is now the most common form of diabetes in pregnancy. The rate of GDM varies tremendously around the world; in some countries it can affect more than one in six or seven pregnancies, in the least affected areas it will affect one in twenty or so. GDM is best understood as a form of temporary T2D, present just during the confines of pregnancy. GDM is rising in all countries in tandem with the increase in T2D everywhere.

For the majority of women affected, GDM brings with it the risk of future T2D – though this can take years to happen. Both GDM and T2D substantially raise the risk of artery disease, and can also impact the health of any child of the pregnancy before birth, after birth, into childhood, and even into adult life – as we'll explain.

To illustrate the issues of T2D, including its impact across generations, we are going to look at what happened to Suzanne. Suzanne's mother had T2D, and then she herself developed GDM. Suzanne and her husband David had been trying for a pregnancy for over three years. Her periods had never been as frequent or regular as they would be for the majority of women. They assumed that fertility might be a problem, but she was still young enough to be patient. When she did become pregnant at the age of thirty-one, her first midwife appointment highlighted her family history and the risk of GDM.

The risk factors for GDM in women are:

- Body mass index over 30.

- GDM in a previous pregnancy.

- Being of South Asian, Black, African Caribbean or Middle Eastern ethnicity.

- Having had a previous baby weighing over 4.5kg (10lb).

- A first degree relative (usually a parent or sibling) with T2D.

What happens to glucose in pregnancy?

In the early months of a healthy pregnancy, a mother's blood glucose is naturally on the low side. Insulin sensitivity is good and glucose is being pushed by insulin into all the right places to help supply energy all around the body. This also helps build up essential fat stores for later in the pregnancy and for breastfeeding.

In the final months of pregnancy, rising hormones from the placenta and the mother cause the reverse situation and insulin resistance dominates. The mother's glucose production 'tap' in the liver is in the on position, and glucose builds in the bloodstream. Insulin resistance (occurring naturally on this occasion) also allows stored fat to break down, so both glucose and fat for fuel are more available in this demanding time for the mother and her baby. This is normal metabolism in pregnancy.

In early pregnancy, a woman's body is tending towards storing fuel. In later pregnancy, it is releasing and delivering fuel – all making perfect sense. If you are one of those women coming into your pregnancy with an already rising insulin and glucose level – at some risk of future T2D – then your pancreas is already working a little harder than normal. In the later stages of pregnancy, the pancreas has to work even harder and insulin production can fail to meet demands, just as it does in T2D outside of pregnancy. Sharply rising blood glucose follows, and that's when GDM develops.

GDM develops like T2D does, with the pregnancy hormones playing a decisive role in pushing susceptible women from an at-risk state to a diabetic state. The diagnostic test for GDM is done around two-thirds of the way through the pregnancy, when the hormonal settings of the pregnancy are allowing blood glucose to rise. The mother's raised blood glucose crossing the placenta causes foetal insulin levels to rise, and too much insulin is not a good start to a baby's life. Hyperglycaemia raises the risk of foetal abnormalities, high blood pressure for the mother and birthing complications such as early or premature labour. A high foetal insulin level leads to the characteristic large baby (macrosomia) of a diabetes pregnancy, in turn raising the likelihood of medical interventions, including assisted delivery and caesarean section.

Elevated levels of glucose in the foetal environment – the bloodstream and amniotic fluid around the baby in the uterus – are known to strongly link with problems for the child, including when they become an adult. Children born of a woman with GDM are more likely to become insulin-resistant, overweight or obese, or even have T2D, by the time they are adults in the reproductive phase of life. This makes the last three months of a diabetes pregnancy critical not just for both baby and mother but also for the health journey of the future child and adult. T2D going into pregnancy is experienced and managed in much the same way as GDM. It is GDM at a higher volume. Insulin resistance is greater, so it's harder to manage blood glucose, but the principles are the same. The difference is that the disease is there before *and* after the pregnancy.

With a family history of T2D, you are several times more likely to develop GDM than usual. Pre-existing insulin resistance might have affected Suzanne's ovaries – affecting fertility and her menstrual cycle. Twenty-six weeks into her pregnancy, Suzanne discovered that she had GDM.

How do people manage their GDM?

GDM and T2D are managed just as they are outside pregnancy, but with more urgency – there are only a few months to get things right. Hyperglycaemia is the target; the connection between the mother's glucose level and the harms we've mentioned is a very strong one, and the need for action is compelling. Blood glucose targets in pregnancy are lower and more women with GDM (and T2D) have medical treatment, especially insulin, to help with that. How many women end up on insulin is hard to say, as country-to-country differences are wide – 50 per cent would not be unusual.

Two weeks of following dietary advice and doing more exercise made little difference to Suzanne's blood glucose, so she was started on metformin and then insulin. Things improved but she was having to monitor her glucose several times a day, along with a daily blood pressure reading. She also had regular scans to track aspects of the pregnancy and the baby's growth.

Having any form of diabetes in pregnancy means making much more time to be looked after, and for looking after yourself – more clinic visits and more tests. Self-monitoring of blood glucose and blood pressure is the norm, whether or not insulin is being used.

We looked at the advice on eating in GDM in several countries, and found that current guidance for pregnancy is more or less standard nutritional and lifestyle advice. Just to re-summarise, eating should be based on unrefined, starchy or grainy carbohydrates, adequate protein and restricted saturated fat. US guidance, for example, has been for 45–65 per cent of daily energy intake to come from carbohydrates – which means around 250–350g per day based on a pregnancy calorie intake of 2,200kcal per day.

There are broadly two ways to manage T2D nutritionally: eat less (energy/food) or eat less carbohydrate. Eating less food in pregnancy is not an option for most women – energy needs are higher in pregnancy, and there are hazards in restricting it. Late pregnancy is a time of natural insulin resistance, and GDM and T2D are insulin-resistant states. Insulin resistance can also be called carbohydrate intolerance, and the term occasionally appears in pregnancy nutritional literature. If a woman is carbohydrate-intolerant, and all pregnant women are to a degree, why base the diet on the one major nutrient which the body struggles to handle? If reducing food energy is not an option then reducing carbohydrate is the only practical option.

It's difficult for authorities to advise eating differently in GDM – they have to support a carbohydrate-based diet to avoid supporting a fat-based diet. Fat avoidance is again at the heart of the problem. Secondly, the relative urgency to control blood glucose within the pregnancy has meant more emphasis on medical therapy. Clinical culture might also be a problem. Doctors, midwives and dieticians are perhaps attuned to diabetes based on the historic management of T1D, which was until recently the role model for managing diabetes in pregnancy. Embedded in that world is the perception that insulin is the way to reliably manage blood glucose, and that ketones are to be avoided. In T1D, the presence of ketones is potentially serious. In T2D/GDM, it is usually not.

Ketones (again)

Ketosis is a term meaning the detectable presence of these small fat-like substances that we all make in the liver, especially during fasts or illnesses. They are detectable in both blood and urine, using simple testing strips. There are three recognised levels of ketosis:

Nutritional ketosis. This is a normal occurrence in pregnancy. Food energy intake is normal, but carbohydrates may have been limited. Blood glucose is normal. In late pregnancy, ketones in the urine may be a sign that a woman's body is preferentially burning fat for fuel. In healthy pregnancy and early infant life, some ketosis is normal.

Starvation ketosis. This might occur in pregnancy if a woman was ill or, for whatever reason, was unable to maintain an adequate food energy intake. Severe morning sickness would be the most common example. Though blood glucose is usually unaffected, this is not good if prolonged, and nutritional deficiencies can occur.

Ketoacidosis. This is a dangerous state, in or out of pregnancy, and nearly always occurs in T1D when insulin is deficient or a person with T1D is severely unwell. Ketone levels and blood glucose are both high. Urgent and intensive treatment is always needed.

Concerns about 'ketosis' stem from the word itself, which people link with ketoacidosis, but the reality is the two are not linked. Nutritional ketosis is normal and not harmful. Low-carbohydrate eating will produce a degree of nutritional ketosis.

On the plus side, current guidance stresses the need for personalised nutritional advice, avoidance of sugar (including restraint with fruits to limit fructose), keeping physically fit and active, and prioritising sleep. These are all positive steps. However, the fact remains that guidelines are still advocating a carbohydrate-based diet for women who are carbohydrate-intolerant, with weak scientific support.

In regular T2D care, it is clinicians (and people with T2D) who are working against the grain of standard advice to bring about change. In the pregnancy world, one such person is the US dietician and diabetes educator Lily Nichols. She makes the point that sensible reductions in carbohydrate, using whole-food diets that are nutritionally dense (plentiful energy), can reduce the need for insulin in pregnancy. They also help prevent or reduce subsequent infant and childhood obesity. Her YouTube presentation on GDM (link in Appendix 3: Resources (for Chapter 9)) is for clinicians but can be followed by those without training. She makes her case with great clarity, simplicity and with the evidence base for what she says. Please watch! In the same appendix is an example wholefood meal plan for GDM, with signposting to further reading on diet if you are pregnant or considering it.

Suzanne gave birth to Chloe successfully. She needed a drip (IV) with insulin to maintain safe blood glucose, and Chloe was a little slow to get breathing. She was breastfed half an hour after emerging, in what Suzanne said was the happiest moment of her life. It was definitely worth all the checks and scans! Chloe weighed 4kg (just under 9lb) – larger than average but not unusual in GDM. Suzanne was able to reduce insulin and stop metformin more or less straight after giving birth. Chloe needed an extra two days in hospital to help with her blood glucose, but then all settled.

Once hormones from the placenta have left her system, a mum's insulin function recovers quickly. In their first day or two, babies can have breathing problems, and sometimes hypoglycaemia. Ideally they need early and frequent breastfeeding, and sometimes extra help. In the uterus they have been exposed to high insulin and glucose levels and, once delivered, their glucose fuel line is literally clamped, causing the blood level to drop. With their own insulin/glucose system up and running, the baby's blood glucose normalises within a day or two.

T2D into the next generation

A child's diet starts before being born – it's their mother's diet – and what a mother eats during her pregnancy can impact the health of her unborn baby. For example, we know that eating too much sugar in pregnancy drives up blood glucose in the baby's environment. The foetal liver gets unneeded practice in turning sugar into fat and an early introduction to insulin resistance. Taste awareness starts in unborn children before those crucial last three months when they are already able to sense sweetness in their fluid surroundings. Is this a very early trigger for the sweet tooth afflicting many of us in later life?

We now know that the foetal environment can imprint on an unborn child the legacy of being exposed to too much sugar. That child is then at higher risk of becoming obese and developing metabolic disease, including T2D, throughout childhood, adolescence and into adult life. But how much sugar is too much? We don't know for sure. If we compare free or added sugar (fructose-containing) in maternal diets to alcohol – its nutritional cousin – then small amounts might be OK. However, what constitutes a small amount? Guidance in the UK recommends eating no more than 30g, or seven tea-spoons, of sugar a day, whereas in the US this is around 50g or twelve teaspoons – a level which research suggests is enough to threaten an unborn child's future health. But these are guides, not what people actually do. Intakes are well in excess of guidance in young adults, indeed in most adults, with the bulk of that sugar hidden in ultra-processed foods and sugary drinks. Most young adults probably consume more sugar than is recommended without being aware. Too much processed food in pregnancy raises an obvious health risk, to the same degree as the more familiar risks of alcohol and smoking.

Early months

After birth, research has shown that breastfed babies whose

mothers eat sugar in excess receive small but potentially harmful levels of fructose in their milk – enough to impact weight and body fat levels in their first few months. Babies, like adults, have no 'machinery' for handling fructose – they turn it into fat just like adults do – and it takes very little to do that, so tiny amounts in breast milk make a difference.

Breastfeeding gives many health benefits, such that current guidelines, including those of the World Health Organization, recommend breastfeeding up to twenty-four months. But is everything in breast milk good? A resounding yes, so long as mum goes easy on sugar-sweetened drinks and processed foods, keeping sugar/fructose low or absent in her milk. Breast milk has the perfect balance of nutrients, as you would expect from nature.

Formula milk and infant foods

Formula milk is tightly regulated in most places, and should be fructose-free, though it's such a complex product that even healthcare professionals can find it difficult to navigate. Relative to breast milk it has slightly less fat and slightly more carbohydrate. The lactose-free/soy-based products should be used with care, as these milks are deficient in galactose (which comes from lactose) which, along with fat, helps to grow baby brains. Infant milk and sugar can confuse as much as sugar in the food world generally. The natural sugar in breast milk is lactose and that should be the case in formula milk too. The only ways that fructose will find its way into an infant's system are from the mother's diet passing into breast milk or a presence in formula milk and infant foods, neither of which should happen – and, of course, parental choice.

Can parents resist giving infants sugar? Not according to some research which suggests that sugary drinks and sweet snacks are commonly started well under two years of age – the minimum age recommended by many authorities. In 2022, research by the British Dental Association highlighted an 'obscene' level of added sugars in infant 'grab-and-go' food pouches, significantly contravening both national and WHO guidance. The food industry clearly knows its market.

Whether it be the dummy dunked in sugar to pacify a fractious baby or unnaturally sweetened early foods to coax fussy infants to eat 'better', the early bond with sugar is well established. In Chapter 6 we talked about processed foods – is formula milk and infant food so much different?

Other research suggests that both bottle feeding (less grip needed than for a nipple) and over-soft infant foods (less chewing needed) can impair palate, airway and jaw development. Structural problems of the mouth and airway can show later as snoring, and crowding or poor alignment of teeth increases the risk of dental problems later. Snoring and obstructive sleep apnoea are strongly linked to metabolic disease, caused in part by disturbed sleep (see Chapter 4).

Suzanne breastfed for three months but stopped due to a combination of fatigue, inconvenience and returning to work. After her postnatal check, she attended for a medical review of her

GDM, and tests showed normal glucose and HbA1c. Like many women, she then missed the recommended further annual reviews of her HbA1c. Her next medical contact was actually five years later when she saw her GP with tummy pains and feelings of tiredness. At this point, her HbA1c was 46mmol/mol (6.4%) – very much at risk but not quite at T2D level.

GDM to T2D

The majority of women with GDM eventually develop T2D, and most do so in the first five years. Every case of GDM is an opportunity to prevent either T2D or further GDM, and yet healthcare systems and women have struggled to connect on this issue. It looks to be slowly improving but regular checks after a GDM pregnancy are definitely worth thinking about.

How long should regular checks continue? The advice would be long-term (maybe lifelong), but it's really a matter of how your health is and how much you want the reassurance. After a GDM pregnancy the risk of future T2D will remain, even into the longer term, so repeating the HbA1c test at intervals and tracking your weight keeps you in control. Why not use your calendar year planner to record a twice-yearly weight and blood test? Or else agree a check and reminder system with your healthcare team.

The UK National Diabetes Audit in 2021 suggested that fewer than one in fifteen women with T2D were 'well prepared' for pregnancy, i.e. having the best possible health and control of blood glucose at the time they became pregnant. This rather bleak snapshot shows just how much needs to be done to raise awareness on health, pregnancy and T2D in younger women and health professionals.

Knowing that you have T2D, and that pregnancy risks all link directly with blood glucose, means working up a plan for managing your diabetes *before* getting pregnant. Ideally, being prepared means the lowest HbA1c achievable and eating in a way that will sustain control through the pregnancy. A diet lower in carbohydrates but not calories, whether it be cutting out sugar, a Mediterranean-style diet, or cutting back on processed food, will help.

If you have T2D and think a future pregnancy a possibility, attempting to put your T2D into remission would be the best approach of all. Delaying pregnancy to get better control makes sense. Very poor control – a HbA1c, say, of around 80mmol/mol (9.5%) – is hazardous, increasing the risk of birth defects, even stillbirth, though that's rare. So the lower the blood glucose (HbA1c) the better.

If you struggle with motivation, remember that your health, diet and diabetes control can affect not just you and the pregnancy outcome, but the long-term health of your future children. If pregnancy is not a choice or would be unwelcome, then access family planning advice from your healthcare practitioner – there is no barrier to contraceptive use in T2D!

When Suzanne was diagnosed with T2D at the age of forty-three, she resolved for all sorts of reasons to put her health at or close to the top of her priorities. This helped her to put her

T2D into remission. She attended regular clinic appointments and had all the routine check-ups that she would have had if her T2D was still active. Her motivation had become more solid. Four years later, Suzanne went back to see her doctor – this time with Chloe, who was now fifteen.

Chloe's story

Being a typical teenager, Chloe didn't want to say a lot! To open things up, her mum said they were both concerned about her getting lower abdominal pains, and that her periods had not yet started (starting at around thirteen is more typical). She had bad acne on her face and appeared overweight. Further enquiry suggested that she could be grumpy, especially around her weight, and her snoring was the butt of family jokes. Her blood pressure was a little raised.

The doctor, aware of Suzanne's medical history, thought it quite likely that Chloe had a related disorder called PCOS (polycystic ovary syndrome), which might have been delaying her periods. PCOS links with insulin resistance and T2D. Chloe's HbA1c was just below the level for being at risk but higher than it should have been. It also links with NAFLD, raised blood pressure, a higher risk of artery disease and sleep problems including snoring. It can be helped by metformin, but as with T2D this would improve but not cure the condition. Reversing PCOS needs the same approach and mindset as for T2D, built around sustainable weight loss. Snoring is a risk factor – perhaps through disturbed sleep and the stress hormone system – for metabolic disease, including T2D.

Six months later, spurred on by the extra incentive of improved skin, Chloe had lost over 10kg (22lb) by sharing her mother's low-carbohydrate diet. Her pains settled, and her blood pressure and HbA1c were normal. Ongoing lower weight and less acne were powerful motivators for Chloe but, as all parents know, it's easy to get derailed as a teenager.

Low-carbohydrate eating, a low- or no-sugar diet and severe calorie restriction can potentially all reverse T2D and related conditions such as PCOS. Keeping it going is the bigger challenge, even more so in younger people. Acne is distressing in the young and there is reasonable evidence of benefit from eating a low-carbohydrate diet. Lowering insulin helps to lower androgens like testosterone (a male hormone which is present in all women at low levels but higher in women with PCOS), which helps skin to be less oily and prone to acne.

Nature or nurture – or both?

For many years, we have been aware of increasing weight and obesity, and the even more alarming rate of an increase in T2D. But if we look at the metabolic family of conditions, and the way *they* are all increasing, things look even worse, if that's possible.

All the conditions in this family are becoming more common – seemingly in step with each other, marching to the same drumbeat, perhaps. The list has increased over the last twenty years, and more could be added:

- Insulin resistance.

- Tummy too big – abdominal fat.

- High blood pressure.

- Non-alcoholic fatty liver disease (NAFLD).

- Blood lipid (fat) changes.

- Artery disease.

- T2D and elevated blood glucose.

- Gout.

- In women – polycystic ovary syndrome (PCOS).

- In men – erectile dysfunction (ED).

- Obstructive sleep apnoea (OSA).

Which are the 'parents' and which are the 'children' in this problem family? For forty years, insulin resistance has been seen as the main driver, but whether it really is a 'single-parent family' remains to be seen. A few people have all of these, and many people have one or other in combination. Put together, more than half of us are in this family somewhere.

Suzanne's mother has T2D, Suzanne herself has T2D, Chloe has PCOS – and both had weight gain and abnormal liver function (suggesting NAFLD). Suzanne had reduced fertility and infrequent periods, and may have had mild PCOS herself. Chloe is at risk of T2D even in her teens.

Cast your eye back to Figures 1.3 and 1.4 in Chapter 1, showing rises over time in T2D and obesity. Why are they rising so fast, especially T2D? Chloe has PCOS and this is rising in exactly the same way. Historically, the rapid spread of a disease has usually been the result of infectious agents, most recently viruses such as influenza or COVID-19, or toxins such as tobacco. The recent surge in T2D has been likened by scientists to that of an exposure; most likely a toxin-like effect, since T2D is not an infectious disease. The phrases 'toxic (food) environment' and 'toxic lifestyle' are used by some. Others think a single substance – sugar (fructose) – might be the main driver of T2D, and we have already acknowledged the research on its harms in pregnancy.

Whether a toxic lifestyle or a single agent is to blame, scientists feel that the surge in T2D and metabolic diseases generally is still unaccountably large. Step in epigenetics.

Epigenetic inheritance

Evolutionary genetics, the process of random mutation and natural selection, changes species (including our own) across many generations – that's hundreds or even thousands of years. Standard genetic theory cannot explain a pandemic of metabolic illness occurring over forty to fifty years, yet undoubtedly our species is changing. We now know that the material of inheritance is of two kinds:

1. Genetic, that is the genes containing our DNA which determine our characteristics in a fixed way, such as whether we have haemophilia or brown eyes, for example.

2. Epigenetic, which is material connected to the genes but not of the DNA itself.

Epigenetic chemistry can influence whether or how genes are expressed. Epigenetic influencers or 'tags' ('labels') can pass quickly through generations, switching genes on and off – producing effects which are reflective of the environment and health of parents and the environment of the unborn child. It's thought too that epigenetic changes can impact a generation beyond, by their effects on the reproductive cells of the unborn child.

Back to Suzanne – and raised blood glucose

Hyperglycaemia can affect three generations at the same time – Suzanne, Chloe not yet born, and Chloe's future children. The impacts on health across four generations (including Suzanne's parents – her mother has T2D) are probably a mixture of genetic and epigenetic effects. The impact of these processes through the male line (Suzanne's own father and her husband, Chloe's father) are not so well known, but we are starting to see that they may be influential too.

Foetal exposure to high glucose causes big babies and increases birth risks. It might also contribute in part to too much fat in infancy. Epigenetic inheritance (possibly from either parent) might then cause the susceptibility to weight gain or T2D as the child grows, and to other metabolic diseases later in life.

If scientists are correct, then reproduction and pregnancy together may be turbo-charging the rise in T2D – a process which seemed to begin as a dietary change across many populations forty or so years ago.

Figure 9.1: Environment, epigenetics and metabolism connect

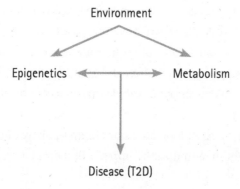

Changes in the environment (in T2D, the food environment) through epigenetics can influence disease rapidly across generations. Metabolism and the epigenome can most definitely influence *each other*, for better or worse. The good news is that, from a T2D perspective, what goes up can come down. The epigenome is susceptible to change. Eating so as to lower insulin and glucose levels, and improving physical fitness, give us a chance of reversing this surge of disease – and improving the health of the next generation.

The key player now in our model family is Chloe. If she can maintain her health and weight, she can minimise epigenetic transmission of the metabolic traits that have clearly come her way. Her own children might remain disease free; the chain *can* be broken.

Epigenetics is really beyond the scope of this book, though an explanation is in Appendix 2: Terminology (for Chapter 9). But epigenetics carries a simple message to all of us about the need to look after and improve the health of children. This need starts in pregnancy but continues through childhood and into early adult life. Even if we are past the usual parenting years, we can still transmit an important verbal, if not epigenetic, message to our children and grandchildren about eating and health. We cannot be complacent or accepting about both rising weight and T2D in the world. If we are to defeat this condition we must look after our children, many of whom are now caught in an unhealthy trap not of their making.

Key points from Chapter 9

- Pregnancy or gestational diabetes (GDM) is akin to T2D, and most women with GDM develop ongoing T2D.

- Progression from GDM to T2D can be prevented, as with T2D itself.

- GDM, once uncommon, now affects 5–20 per cent of pregnancies around the world.

- Insulin is commonly used in GDM to control hyperglycaemia.

- Reducing carbohydrates (not calories) in the diet is an option for managing GDM and can reduce the need for insulin.

- In T2D, controlling hyperglycaemia (HbA1c) or reversing the T2D is best done *before* pregnancy.

- The health of children born in GDM and T2D pregnancies is potentially affected before birth, and after pregnancy into infancy, childhood and beyond.

- Reversing the upward trend in weight and metabolic disease in children and younger adults could limit the epigenetic 'spread' of T2D.

- Teenage girls and younger women need help to become more T2D-aware.

Looking after your psychological wellbeing: getting started

FAST – dealing with tension, stress, low mood and anxiety part 1

Type 2 diabetes doesn't just affect people physically; it is very likely to affect you emotionally too. Living with T2D isn't straightforward, especially at first. It can feel overwhelming. This is why we are dedicating Chapters 10 and 11 to psychological wellbeing and strategies you can use to tackle psychological difficulties related to your T2D. In this chapter, we'll look at the emotional impact of a T2D diagnosis as well as how it can feel to live with T2D in the longer term. We'll teach you how to clearly define your problem, before working towards realistic and achievable goals. We'll cover two well-tested strategies to help you with your problems; we'll take a similar line in Chapter 11 when we look at how to manage negative thoughts, ruminations and worries.

Let's start with the emotional impact of being diagnosed with and living with T2D. Feelings can include: low mood, worry, anxiety, anger and other upsetting emotions. It may feel sometimes that your life has been taken over and is controlled by T2D. Others around you can be affected too. It is important to remember that you are not alone in having these feelings. Research shows that people with a diagnosis of T2D are more likely to experience mental health issues such as depression – but that doesn't mean you can't do anything about it. In the first two sections of the book we emphasised how everything connects in T2D. Eating well, being more active and getting a good night's sleep all help with how you feel, both in your mind and body. In this chapter and Chapter 11, we will look at what else you can do to help with the emotional side of T2D including looking at your thoughts, feelings and behaviours.

In Chapter 1 we asked what thoughts and feelings you had when you were first diagnosed with T2D. Now is a good time to look at those notes, or to make a note of your thoughts and feelings now so you can try some of the strategies in this chapter.

Talking about your T2D. Talking to people close to you about your feelings around T2D is a good idea but it's not always easy to do. Who do you confide in? What do you say? You might worry about burdening someone else with your problems. You might not even want to talk to someone about it. What we know is that talking can help, not just for the person with T2D but for the people close to them too. There are often lots of people to talk to about it, such as family, friends, your health-care team, diabetes organisations and other people in a similar position to you, including support groups. Consider looking at what is available in your area.

Coping with a diagnosis of T2D. For many people, receiving a diagnosis of T2D comes as a shock. It's not unusual to experience disbelief, anger, anxiety or distress – and occasionally relief to discover what is wrong – especially if, like Cassie, the worry was about cancer. As with any shock, these feelings usually ease after a while as you get on with life and adapt to the diagnosis. Unfortunately, that's not always the case for everyone and if you are one of the many people who experience ongoing emotional difficulties following a diagnosis of T2D, this chapter and Chapter 11 may well help you.

First we will focus on depression, then T2D distress.

Depression is incredibly common in the general population. In fact, according to the World Health Organization, around one in twenty people suffer from depression, which increases over the age of sixty. People with a long-term physical health condition are two to three times more likely to develop depression. This is perhaps not surprising given how difficult it can be to live with conditions like T2D on a day-by-day basis – it is always there and that can be exhausting. It can get you down.

Depression (and many other mental health problems) sometimes genuinely precede T2D, and we now know that a stressed brain triggers hormone and nerve responses which can lead to insulin resistance. Not everyone with depression experiences the same symptoms but we've included some of the more common ones in Figure 10.1. If you experience five or more of the symptoms highlighted in bold in Figure 10.1 for more than two weeks, and at least one of the symptoms is either depressed mood or loss of interest or pleasure, you should visit your doctor.

Figure 10.1: Common symptoms of depression

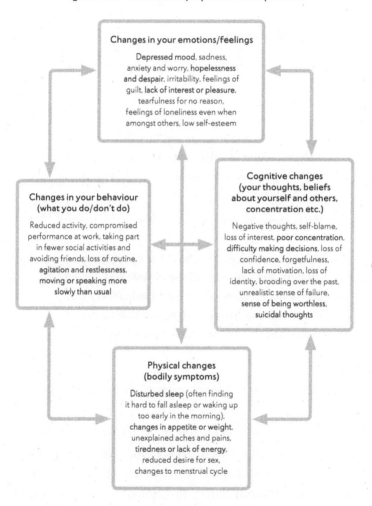

Changes in your emotions/feelings

Depressed mood, sadness, anxiety and worry, hopelessness and despair, irritability, feelings of guilt, lack of interest or pleasure, tearfulness for no reason, feelings of loneliness even when amongst others, low self-esteem

Cognitive changes (your thoughts, beliefs about yourself and others, concentration etc.)

Negative thoughts, self-blame, loss of interest, poor concentration, difficulty making decisions, loss of confidence, forgetfulness, lack of motivation, loss of identity, brooding over the past, unrealistic sense of failure, sense of being worthless, suicidal thoughts

Changes in your behaviour (what you do/don't do)

Reduced activity, compromised performance at work, taking part in fewer social activities and avoiding friends, loss of routine, agitation and restlessness, moving or speaking more slowly than usual

Physical changes (bodily symptoms)

Disturbed sleep (often finding it hard to fall asleep or waking up too early in the morning), changes in appetite or weight, unexplained aches and pains, tiredness or lack of energy, reduced desire for sex, changes to menstrual cycle

The greater the number of symptoms, the more likely the depression is to markedly interfere with your day-to-day functioning like going to work and looking after children.

> ### Pause for thought
>
> Take a pause and think through whether you are experiencing any of these symptoms. Try to use a diagram like Figure 10.1. By doing this, it will mean you can start to consider how each symptom area may be impacting your life and how they interact with each other. It will also help when we come on to problem statements and setting goals a bit later in the chapter.
>
> If you think you are depressed please speak to your healthcare team, who will be able to talk to you about how to access psychological treatment and support, and what is available in your area. If your doctor offers you antidepressant medication there is no need to worry about how it will affect any diabetes medication you are taking – it won't.

When some people feel very depressed, they can think that life is no longer worth living and may make plans to end their life. If things ever get so bad for you and you have thoughts about ending your life, it is vital to get help right away. In Appendix 3: Resources (for Chapter 10) there are details of support agencies that you can contact twenty-four hours a day. Get in touch with your doctor and your healthcare team urgently. It is crucial that you get help. It is important to remind yourself that you will not always feel this way and that there are things you can do to feel better and to live a good life with T2D.

Quality of life. A diagnosis of T2D can negatively impact quality of life and socialising with others, which can affect mental wellbeing not just in the short term but in the long term too. But this does not have to be the case. It is important not to reduce time spent with friends and family, attending clubs and groups that you have previously enjoyed or other activities with people outside the home. Keep going out and live your life!

Depression, anxiety and distress – similarities and differences. Sometimes the symptoms of anxiety or depression are not so bad or prolonged that we need to see them as separate problems, but we should acknowledge their presence in long-term conditions like T2D; an extra 'diagnosis' might not be needed or helpful. You could argue that it is natural to feel low or worried when diagnosed with a challenging illness. Perhaps it is better to normalise the experience of distress in long-term physical health conditions – which is where diabetes distress comes in.

Diabetes distress is the term used for the negative emotional response that people have to living with T2D. In this section, we will be looking at diabetes distress but not necessarily as a mental health disorder. Hopefully you'll feel that the term diabetes distress accurately reflects the challenge of adjusting to having T2D. This includes the emotions a person feels on receiving the diagnosis of T2D and also as a reaction to the challenging life changes that the diagnosis brings, of ongoing daily self-management and the emotions a person may feel around possible long-term complications. The distress also includes any impact the diagnosis may have on social aspects of life. This includes feelings of stigma, dealing with other people's reactions – such as discrimination or a lack of under-standing – and also any financial implications, such as getting to and from routine hospital appointments, travel and health insurance, etc., as well as worries about the future. Some peo-ple face work difficulties too.

Like depression and anxiety, diabetes distress does not happen to everyone and can go up and down over time. It can be at its worst at diagnosis, at times in life when other challenges are getting in the way that lead to heightened stress (divorce, losing a loved one, moving house, etc.), making major lifestyle changes, and/or any worsening of symptoms or diagnosis of complications.

Suzanne lost her way with her health when she moved house, and from being at risk of diabetes, she developed full-blown T2D – her stresses made it hard for her to prioritise a healthy lifestyle.

Distress in the context of T2D is defined as a negative emotional reaction to the wide range of stressors related to the condition, including diagnosis and self-management challenges. Diabetes distress can include low mood, anxiety, guilt and shame. These negative emotions signal that something is wrong and requires attention, which is no bad thing in many ways as it is a call to action. So how do you know whether your diabetes distress is a problem to tackle or to leave alone? It is really down to the severity of the distress, how long it lasts, and the impact on your functioning and ability to live your life.

What's the difference between diabetes distress and depression? There are some overlapping symptoms between the two but diabetes distress is different to a formal diagnosis of depression. Diabetes distress is an expected reaction to having T2D whereas depression goes beyond the T2D to be more about life in general, and can precede a diagnosis of T2D, like it did for Colin. When diabetes distress is long-lasting and severe, it may lead to depression. Evidence is emerging suggesting that being pessimistic about having T2D and its treatment along with low adherence to treatment are linked to greater symptoms of depression and anxiety.

How many people with T2D get diabetes distress? About one in six people with T2D experience diabetes distress, rather more in those who are on insulin, so it is very common. A person is more likely to experience diabetes distress if they are experiencing difficulties with T2D self-management (e.g. reduced physical activity, eating less healthily, not adhering to medication as prescribed, not monitoring blood glucose if and when they should), and a higher HbA1c may result. This is not to say that a person who has good T2D self-management and optimal HbA1c can't experience diabetes distress – they can.

Mental health problems are common so you may have already had a problem in this respect before the T2D diagnosis. Colin had been troubled with depression for some time before his T2D diagnosis and the roots of both may have been intertwined. Coping with T2D and likely additional diabetes distress made his depression worse and he found the whole thing exhausting. Colin sought professional help for his depression and received a full course of cognitive behavioural therapy (CBT) which helped him enormously, and it was also a helpful way in to managing sexual dysfunction, which helped his mood even further.

Having a greater sense of control over T2D is linked with better problem-solving, seeking out more help and advice, and simply engaging more with the condition. Not feeling in control is linked with a less successful coping style such as avoidance (we will come back to avoidance later). Amongst the biggest causes of diabetes distress are lifestyle changes. Let's look at how CBT can help.

We will focus on the key strategies that are most likely to be of use to you. We will show how some of our case examples used these strategies to help them adjust to diagnosis and learned how to live with T2D. The aim is to relieve the source of your distress by using tried and tested approaches. We will look at how aspects of a T2D diagnosis can lead to distress and effective coping strategies to lessen these negative effects. We want you to have a greater sense of control over the diagnosis and the stressors linked to it and help you to develop a tool bag of techniques that you can use when you need them.

In Chapter 8, we looked at self-monitoring and the idea of being more of a self-manager. We explained how it can help to align your expectations with what's reasonably *achievable*, especially the timescale for experiencing a change. It can feel frustrating at times when things are slow to move, especially when trying to lose weight – we will talk about goal-setting shortly. We also made the point that sometimes we can be too tolerant of failure. If something doesn't work and has had a long enough trial, it's time to rethink!

Self-management can seem different depending on where you are in your T2D journey. Things can feel overwhelming at the outset after a new diagnosis. You can be expected to stick to treatment plans, make necessary lifestyle changes and navigate what can feel like complicated health systems and consultations with new healthcare professionals. At the same time, you might be feeling unwell as well as low or anxious. Then through time, you become more familiar with what's required. Things can feel less stressful but it's still important to keep a check on how things are going (what's helping, what's not), especially if you experience a change in symptoms or new guidance from your healthcare team. There is always something to think about.

The prospect of a reversal of T2D brings a new challenge and even if it is not possible to fully reverse T2D, it is most definitely possible to improve it with the sort of changes we covered in the first two sections of the book. Managing expectations has now moved on. Each person needs to be able to form a view with the help of their team – just what is the potential for your own T2D to be improved? Being in control and self-managing will then be shaped by this new knowledge and a new aiming point. Even some simple self-monitoring can help and simplify things rather than complicating your life.

Ted was the least likely of people to become involved in self-monitoring. He made a few dietary changes but preferred to leave most things to his healthcare practitioner. However, after his T2D diagnosis and meeting more people with the condition, he decided to try monitoring his blood pressure at home. To his surprise, he took to this like a duck to water. He enjoyed the feeling of participation, and the sense that he knew his blood pressure was OK – *he* was checking it. He didn't need to wait anxiously for it to be measured in the clinic.

Over the remainder of this chapter we are going to look at strategies that can help with mental wellbeing. First, it can be helpful to take stock of where you are at by defining exactly what the problem is and setting some goals.

Getting started: identifying the problem(s) with your mood

Identifying the problem is an important starting point. Breaking down difficulties into problem statements can help focus the mind on what needs to happen to make things better. A problem statement is a summary of your difficulties in a nutshell. There are three key elements to a problem statement and they are:

- The trigger.

- The symptoms (emotional, physical, cognitive, behavioural).

- The consequences or impact.

Problem statements tend to contain words such as 'my problem is', 'leading to' and 'as a result'. Let's look at some examples to give an idea of how to come up with your problem statement.

Cassie's problem statement – a few months after her diagnosis. 'I was relieved that I didn't have cancer, but it was still a shock to be told I had T2D. My main problem is still feeling devastated by the diagnosis. This has led to me feeling angry and upset with myself, and I get tense and shaky when I think about it. I believe that I am a failure for getting T2D and avoid talking about it due to embarrassment and shame. As a result, I see my friends less and feel more lonely and down. My future seems more uncertain now and I worry that I won't be able to stay in control of my health.'

Notice the trigger – the diagnosis of T2D. Symptoms: relief initially, then anger and upset, embarrassment and shame (emotional); tense and shaky (physical); 'I am a failure' (cognitive); avoiding talking about it (behavioural). Consequences: lonely and down and feeling that the future is uncertain.

Benjamin's problem statement – four years after diagnosis. 'My main problem is coming to terms with the changes that T2D is making to my life. I feel sad and find it difficult to sleep for thinking about it. This has led me to worry that I will end up on insulin which would be the end of my job. It feels like life can never be good again. I hide things from everyone, so people think I'm OK. I don't go out so much with friends these days as I have to steer the conversation away from my diabetes. As a result, I am becoming a bit more isolated.'

Notice the trigger – the changes T2D is making to life. Symptoms: sad and worried (emotional); difficulty sleeping (physical); 'life can never be good again' (cognitive); seeing friends less (behavioural). Consequences: more isolated.

Nandita's problem statement – ten years after diagnosis. 'My main problem is sticking to the guidance for my T2D. This has led me to feel anxious and resentful, and I get headaches and body tension when I deviate from what I should be doing. It feels like I can never be truly happy again. I get obsessed with biscuits and just have to have one which often leads to more. As a result, my blood glucose is all over the place and I am worried about the effect this will have on my long-term health.'

Notice the trigger – sticking to T2D guidance. Symptoms: anxious and resentful (emotional); headaches and body tension (physical); 'I can never be truly happy again' (cognitive); comfort-eating biscuits (behavioural). Consequences: erratic blood glucose and worries about future health.

All these problem statements have a theme around T2D but are all different in terms of the problem, the symptoms and the consequences. Your problem statement is likely to be different too. The last step is to rate the problem statement on a scale of 0–100, to indicate how severe it is currently (see Figure 10.2).

Figure 10.2: Problem scale 0–100

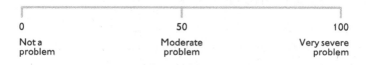

0	50	100
Not a problem	Moderate problem	Very severe problem

Exercise

Your problem statement

Try to come up with your own problem statement. The problem is the one that causes the most disruption to your life and is usually the most severe. Use the prompts to help: trigger, symptoms (emotional, physical, cognitive, behavioural), and consequences or impact. Then rate your problem using the scale provided. If your rating is very low, yet you feel that the problem is actually more severe, spend a bit of time adjusting your problem statement so it truly captures your problem. Try to come back to your problem statement every now and again (perhaps every couple of weeks or so) to track any improvement as you work your way through tackling your problems.

Pause for thought

Now you have come up with your problem statement, do you have a better idea of why your problem persists? By looking at triggers, symptoms and consequences, you are likely to have formulated some ideas not only about what your problem is but what is keeping it going. This understanding of what is keeping your problem going is important in order to make changes. Next step, goals!

SMART goals

We know that setting goals is a good way to work towards positive change to help the problems you've identified. The best kinds of goals are simple and trackable, making it easy for you to check your progress – they are SMART! Having **s**pecific, **m**easurable, **a**chievable, **r**elevant and **t**imely T2D self-management goals provides a useful framework for measuring your progress in better managing your T2D.

Goals should be things that you want to do – maybe you used to do them but stopped – and should align with your problem statement and your values (more about values later). Self-management goals are particularly useful here. Make sure that your goals are not vague (e.g. 'be less upset about my T2D', 'be happier') and always explicit and clear. This means that goals are best set in easily measured terms so it is obvious whether they are achieved or not (e.g. 'go to the cinema once a week with friends' rather than 'do normal stuff again'). This helps make them specific and measurable. They should be achievable so there's no point in aiming for something that you are unlikely to be able to do. To go from being inactive to running a marathon in three months is not achievable or realistic. Keep your goals relevant – they should directly align with your problem statement and therefore be relevant to *you*. They should be realistic too – it is not realistic to expect dramatic weight loss within a week of lifestyle changes. Being timely is important – think about when you want to achieve the goal and how you are going to do it. No matter how ambitious your goal is, you need to set a realistic timeline for it.

One last word on goals: it is best to write goals positively so that it is clear what you are working towards, rather than what you want to stop doing (e.g. 'go to the pub twice a week for an hour with my partner' rather than 'stop moping around the house').

Here are some examples of SMART goals:

- Engage in physical activity/exercise for at least twenty minutes five days a week.

- Take my T2D medication every day as prescribed.

- Meet a friend socially at least once a week for a couple of hours.

- Eat lunch with work colleagues at least three times a week.

- Cook own dinner/supper/tea from scratch at least four times a week.

Now you have your problem statement and goals, we are ready to look at how to tackle the problem. When diabetes distress is an issue there are some specific interventions which can help. We shall look at these shortly. We need to: identify the T2D stressors, explore your thoughts and beliefs around T2D and its treatment, identify any beliefs that are inaccurate and decide what parts of the stressors may require some support to make a change. Interventions focused on managing T2D stressors, although helpful, are unlikely to be enough on their own to address diabetes distress. While channelling energy into T2D self-management is vital, you will also need energy to focus on dealing with unhelpful emotions. Sometimes people initially experience diabetes distress and then go on to develop a mental health problem which requires direct attention, and this is where CBT can really help too. We'll help you tackle some of the things you might experience, including:

- Avoiding doing things that can lead to unpleasant thoughts and emotions.

- Avoiding uncomfortable thoughts, feelings and physical sensations.

- Heightened self-focus so that you notice things about yourself more.

- Ruminating or going over and over things – worrying much of the time.

Here we'll concentrate on helping you to reduce actions (behaviours) which are avoidant, and the rest we'll deal with in Chapter 11.

Tackling behavioural avoidance

When feeling depressed, anxious, under stress or angry, it is natural to want to do less and to withdraw from activities that were previously enjoyed. This can seem like the best way to cope when life feels overwhelming. The problem with this short-term response is that it can make things worse in the long term. So, for example, not seeing friends (to avoid anticipated stress) can lead to even lower mood and reduces opportunities to experience pleasure. In this section, we will encourage you to try to increase your activity and use problem-solving to tackle life issues.

Here's why increasing activity levels in diabetes distress and depression is helpful. When you feel sad, preoccupied and lacking motivation, you start to do less. You can lack the drive to get going and may believe that you need to get better before you can get back to your old routines. In fact, research suggests the opposite. Making a start and pushing yourself through that barrier of inactivity can begin to lift your mood, reduce negative feelings and make you feel physically better. We know that it's likely to help the brain chemistry but it also improves self-esteem and a sense of having some control over how you feel.

This 'outside-in' approach is called behavioural activation and we think it can have a big impact on T2D, especially if mood is a barrier to you looking after yourself.

Behavioural activation

Getting started. We are going to start with establishing a baseline of your activity. You can do this by completing a daily monitoring diary like the one in Table 10.1 (a blank version can be found in Appendix 3: Resources (for Chapter 10)) for a few days to check exactly what you are doing. Monitoring diaries break each day of the week down into hourly blocks of time.

Stage 1: Establish a baseline by monitoring activity level. This is a crucial first step. It establishes what you are doing and not doing each day right at the start, before making changes. Record what you are doing on an hour-by-hour basis in the daily monitoring diary. It can be good to do this for up to a week. As you write down what you are doing each hour, rate each activity for level of importance/sense of achievement (0–10) and level of enjoyment/pleasure (0–10). The higher the scores, the greater the sense of achievement and pleasure experienced. For example, eating a snack may give a sense of enjoyment but not much in the way of achievement. Planning low-carb/calorie meals for a week is important and may give a sense of achievement, but it gives little pleasure. By doing this, important learning takes place about the impact activities have on feelings of achievement and pleasure.

Monitoring activities also helps identify activities that occur too often and those that do not occur often enough. For example, Nandita's diary showed that she is spending much of her time sitting watching TV. By examining the diary, she was able to think about how sitting watching TV impacts her mood.

The optimum time for completing the monitoring diary. Try to complete the diary as close as possible to completing the activity to ensure that what you have done is not forgotten. It also helps make ratings more accurate. However, if this isn't possible, try to make a note at three-hourly intervals (or other regular time points) throughout the day.

Why is establishing a baseline a good idea? Sometimes we don't really notice what we are doing throughout the day. Recording what you've actually done for a week can provide a rich source of information and can be used to target areas that are most likely to help you. It is worth noting, though, that keeping a diary like this *can* feel tedious, so it is understandable if you struggle to do a full week. Any information is better than none but do give it your best shot!

Nothing is too mundane to record. Do record inactive activities such as 'lying in bed' or 'sitting looking out of the window' as this information is just as valuable, especially if this is a time when you are more likely to ruminate/worry/feel down. For example, Nandita would lie in bed staring at the ceiling thinking about her T2D, which led to distress and worry. Table 10.1 shows her partially completed daily monitoring diary. You will see that Nandita has given a rating of her overall sense of her mood for the day.

Table 10.1: Nandita's partially completed daily
monitoring diary

Daily monitoring diary			
Time of Day	Activity	Enjoyment/ Pleasure Rating 0–10	Importance/ Achievement Rating 0–10
6–7 a.m.	Asleep		
7–8 a.m.	Awake but still in bed	0	0
8–9 a.m.	Lying staring at the ceiling		
9–10 a.m.	Same		
10–11 a.m.	Same		
11 a.m.– 12 p.m.	Got up. Took metformin tablet, then coffee and cereal, then two slices of toast with jam	6	1
12–1 p.m.	Watched TV	3	2
1–2 p.m.	Friend popped round and had lunch together	5	4
2–3 p.m.	Bath	7	4
3–4 p.m.	Went back to bed	0	0
4–5 p.m.	Took metformin then ate a sandwich and four chocolate biscuits	5	2
5–6 p.m.	Watched TV	0	1
6–7 p.m.	Friend rang	4	1

7–8 p.m.	Watched TV	2	0
8–9 p.m.	Same		
9–10 p.m.	Same		
10–11 p.m.	Had nightly insulin injection, then had two slices of toast when watching TV	4	0
11 p.m.– 12 a.m.	Went to bed but couldn't sleep	0	0
12–1 a.m.	Asleep		
1–2 a.m.	Asleep		
2–3 a.m.	Awake, watched TV in bed. Got up and made a cup of tea and a slice of toast	0	0
3–4 a.m.	Awake, watched TV in bed	0	0
4–5 a.m.	Asleep		
5–6 a.m.	Asleep		
Overall mood for the day:			2.5

If you think behavioural activation could be helpful for you, use the daily monitoring diary in Appendix 3: Resources (for Chapter 10) to keep a record of your activities for one week.

Stage 2: Identifying life areas, values and activities. Once you have established your current level of activity and how that activity is impacting your mood, the next step is to think about what changes need to be made to what you are doing on a day-to-day basis. To do this, it's most helpful to think about

how you value things in the important personal areas of your
life – such as those shown in Table 10.2.

Table 10.2: Life areas

Relationships	Forming and maintaining close relationships with others, including family, friends and/or romantic partner.
Education/Career/Work	Formal education or self-learning such as reading books, and your current job, or finding work.
Recreation/Interests	Leisure time, having fun or relaxing, volunteering.
Mind/Body/Spirituality	Physical and mental health, religion and/or spirituality.
Regular Responsibilities	Obligations and respon-sibilities to others and to your belongings. This could include things like cleaning, tidying, shopping, cooking, looking after home/children, paying bills.

Once you have considered different life areas, the next step is to
identify your values in each of these areas. A value is an ideal,

quality or strong belief in your way of living. Ask yourself, what is important to me about each of these life areas? What are you striving to be in each life area? What is it about that life area that is important to you? The value will be important and personal to you, and can be very different to the values of other people you know. Here is Nandita's completed form.

Table 10.3: My values: Nandita

Relationships	Being a caring and loving wife, and a good friend.
Education/Career/Work	Being happy in my retirement.
Recreation/Interests	Being an active person and appreciative of the arts.
Mind/Body/Spirituality	Being as healthy as possible inside and out.
Regular Responsibilities	Be more in control of my diabetes.

Now it's your turn. Think through your values and how you want to live your life in each life area. Make a note of what you want to achieve in each area of your values. You can find a blank form for this in Appendix 3: Resources (for Chapter 10) or simply make a note. Looking at Nandita's values might be helpful. What are the similarities and differences to your own? This is an important step so please don't miss it out.

Stage 3: Activity selection and ranking. The next step is to choose activities for each value by breaking down values into specific activities. An activity is something you do that can be observed, such as going for a walk. Thinking happier thoughts is not an activity. Try to select a mix of easy and difficult activities which can include some that you are already doing. These activities don't need to cost money (e.g. going for a walk or calling a friend). What we will do next is focus on these activities. Try to ensure that your chosen activities are enjoyable or important to you, or both! Have a look at Nandita's list of activities:

Life area: Relationships

Value: Caring for others.

Activities: Have a night out with my husband at least once a fortnight.

Phone my daughter at least twice a week.

Spend time with friends at least once a week.

Life area: Education/Career/Work

Value: Being happy in my retirement.

Activities: Learn to use music-composing software on my laptop.

Volunteer to assist at my old school.

Do voluntary work – I know the food bank is looking for helpers.

Life area: Recreation/Interests

Value: Being active and creative.

Activities: Go for a walk for at least twenty minutes every day.

Swim twice a week.

Go to an art gallery, exhibition or concert at least once a month.

Life area: Mind/Body/Spirituality

Value: Being physically and mentally healthy.

Activities: Do a relaxation session for fifteen minutes every day.

Follow the eating plan I agreed with the dietician.

Attend all my health appointments.

Life area: Regular responsibilities

Value: Being in better control of my diabetes.

Activities: Check my blood glucose once a day.

Check my feet once a week.

Eat nuts instead of biscuits.

It might be that you want to focus on just one or two life areas, but it is often most helpful to include a wide range of life areas. Activities should be observable and measurable and vary in difficulty, with only a small number that could be classed as long-term goals (e.g. be free of T2D). In total there should be fifteen activities. The next step is to list them in any order in an activity list, then rank them from 1–15 from least difficult to hardest. A copy of a blank activity list can be found in Appendix 3: Resources (for Chapter 10).

Table 10.4: Nandita's activity list

Activity list

Instructions: List your desired fifteen activities and rank them in order of difficulty from 1 = least difficult to 15 = most difficult.

Activity	Indicate level of difficulty (1–15)
Have a night out with my husband at least once a fortnight	2
Phone my daughter at least twice a week	1
Spend time with friends at least once a week	12
Work on the composing software at least twice a week	6
Contact school about voluntary assistant work	8
Speak to friend who works in the food bank	3

Go for a walk for at least twenty minutes every day	7
Swim twice a week	9
Go to an art gallery, exhibition or concert at least once a month	4
Do a relaxation session for fifteen minutes every day	5
Follow the eating plan I agreed with the dietician	15
Attend all my health appointments	10
Check my blood glucose once a day	14
Check my feet once a week	11
Eat nuts instead of biscuits	13

Pause for thought

What do you notice about Nandita's activity list? Nandita tended to find that activities related to her family were less difficult than ones related to managing her T2D. Toughest activities don't need to wait until the others are under way. Rather, it can be useful to break some more difficult tasks into small steps. See the next section on how to do that.

EXERCISE

Your activity list

It's your turn now. Use the activity list in Appendix 3: Resources (for Chapter 10) to make your own activity list and rank your activities in order of difficulty.

Stage 4: Scheduling activities and grading of tasks. The next step is to work towards increasing activity by using the list to plan activities linked to your values. The emphasis is always on attempting the planned activity and not on its successful completion. Although it is often best to start with the easiest activities, some may be more urgent than others, so it is worth looking to see whether the activities related to health that are rated as more difficult can be broken down into smaller steps. For instance, Nandita rated following her agreed eating plan the most difficult, and it is easy to see why this may be the case. But there are various steps that can be taken that may be rated as easier to do from the outset. She decided to focus on cutting out snacks and biscuits first, then build up to tackling main meals one at a time, starting with lunch.

The same diary used for monitoring can be used for planning activities for each coming week. The aim is to increase activity, re-establish routine, and establish new routines linked to T2D as needed and to maximise levels of achievement and pleasure. Planning activities in advance can help alleviate problems of indecision and putting things off. Some people get stuck at this point, because they find it hard enough to do the things they are currently doing, let alone increase their activity levels. If this happens to you, remember that we are using an 'outside-in' approach. Use your monitoring diary to guide when activities should be planned.

The idea is to write a plan of activities for the coming week, which you then follow. Although behaviour is the focus of this approach, thoughts and emotions are not ignored. Try to keep an eye on them too, as you are likely to notice an improvement in these areas as your activity increases.

Make sure your plan is flexible enough to allow for unforeseen circumstances (i.e. there is no obligation to walk in heavy rain!). Missed activities can be rescheduled for another time. Nandita sometimes forgot to check her feet on the usual day, but the reminder app on her phone prompted her to do it within the following week. Planning tasks in this way increases the chances of them being carried out, and you spend time on the things that matter to you whilst also having a sense of pleasure and/or achievement.

Although you might be keen to make strides in a particular area, it may not always be possible to dive in and do that particular activity right away. Try to ensure that only a small number are long-term goals (e.g. run a half marathon!). A copy of a blank weekly activity schedule can be found in Appendix 3: Resources (for Chapter 10).

Table 10.5: Nandita's activity schedule for the coming week

Activity schedule

Instructions: Please write in each box for every hour of the day:
Activity, Achievement (A = 0–10) and Pleasure (P = 0–10)

Time	Monday	Tuesday	Wednesday	Thursday	Friday	Saturday	Sunday
6–7 a.m.							
7–8 a.m.	Check blood glucose	Check blood glucose	Check blood glucose	Check blood glucose	Check blood glucose	Check blood glucose	Check blood glucose
8–9 a.m.	Take medication with breakfast	Take medication with breakfast	Take medication with breakfast	Take medication with breakfast	Take medication with breakfast	Take medication with breakfast	Take medication with breakfast
9–10 a.m.	Talk to Sarah on the phone			Talk to Sarah on the phone			
10–11 a.m.	Go for a 20-minute walk	Go for a 20-minute walk	Go for a 20-minute walk	Go for a 20-minute walk	Attend health appointment	Go for a 20-minute walk	Go for a 20-minute walk
11 a.m.–12 p.m.				Do some gardening for 20-minutes	Attend health appointment		
12–1 p.m.							
1–2 p.m.	Meal	Meal	Meal	Meal	Meal	Meal	Meal
2–3 p.m.	Work on composing software			Work on composing software			

3–4 p.m.	Relaxation session	Relaxation session	Relaxation session	Relaxation session	Relaxation session	Relaxation session	Relaxation session
4–5 p.m.							Check feet
5–6 p.m.	Take medication with meal	Take medication with meal	Take medication with meal	Take medication with meal	Take medication with meal	Take medication with meal	Take medication with meal
6–7 p.m.							
7–8 p.m.				Eat out with David			
8–9 p.m.							
9–10 p.m.	Insulin injection	Insulin injection	Insulin injection	Insulin injection	Insulin injection	Insulin injection	Insulin injection
10–11 p.m.	Go to bed	Go to bed	Go to bed	Go to bed	Go to bed	Go to bed	
11 p.m.–12 a.m.						Go to bed	Go to bed
12–1 a.m.							
1–2 a.m.							
2–3 a.m.							
3–4 a.m.							
4–5 a.m.							
5–6 a.m.							

EXERCISE

Planning activities

Plan at least one activity a day for the next week. Try to include things that are likely to give a sense of achievement and/or enjoyment. Make a note in a blank activity schedule of when you will do them. Use a daily monitoring diary to rate how each activity goes in terms of enjoyment and achievement. Both the activity schedule and the daily monitoring diary are in Appendix 3: Resources (for Chapter 10) which can be used for this purpose. See Table 10.5 for Nandita's plan for the week.

Grading tasks

At times, it can be helpful to break some activities down into smaller, more manageable steps. This can be done by using time limits rather than completion of a full task – 'spend ten minutes gardening' as opposed to 'clear the garden of weeds'. Also, the level of difficulty of the activity can be graded, i.e. going for a ten-minute walk and building this up prior to spending an afternoon out with a walking group.

Beware of setting over-ambitious targets that increase the chances of failure, which will only serve to make you feel worse. Grading tasks increases the chance of success. The aim is to gradually re-establish routine and, by grading activities, you can progressively get back into doing the things you used to do prior to the diagnosis of T2D, which will ultimately improve your mood.

Activities can vary hugely depending on your current level of activity. An early task may be to go to bed to sleep each night rather than to sleep in an armchair, or it may be about getting out of bed earlier in the day (e.g. get up at 8 a.m. each day rather than midday), cooking a healthy meal, phoning a friend, or going for a fifteen-minute walk, etc.

Gradual introduction of concentration tasks. It's hard to concentrate when you feel distressed or your mood is low; you might stop reading or have difficulty concentrating on TV programmes that you previously enjoyed. Levels of concentration can gradually be increased with practice. It could be about opting to watch the main items on the news, reading a few pages of a book or one article from a newspaper. Each of these tasks can be progressively increased as concentration improves. Even if you were previously used to regularly reading a book in a day, being able to read a single chapter may take considerable effort and this achievement should be rated accordingly.

Focus on life problems. If you have stopped addressing important practicalities that need to be dealt with (paying bills, following important medical advice, etc.) these can be dealt with using this approach. Health-related tasks – addressing inattention to wellbeing – are particularly important for people with T2D.

Continuation. Keep adding activities over the coming weeks until you are able to regularly complete your fifteen activities. You can even add other activities as you progress if you feel you have time in your week for them. Keep hold of your completed daily activity diaries so that you can chart your progress with time. Comparing diaries from week to week can be very encouraging as you can see how much more active you are becoming. It is not practical, nor is it necessary, for a diary such as this to be kept up long-term. When you stop using the diary is entirely up to you. You might reduce it to entries of important events only and then gradually stop it altogether.

Reflection. If you try behavioural activation for a few weeks, use the following questions to reflect on the experience:

- Were you able to make changes to your activity? If so, what were the changes you made?

- What was the impact of each of them?

- Were there any surprises? If so, what were they?

- What conclusions can you draw from increasing the activities you engage in? What will you continue to do from now on?

Problem-solving

Problem-solving is a straightforward and effective way of finding solutions to everyday life problems. It is a particularly useful approach for tackling practical aspects of all sorts of problems including those related to T2D.

When feeling overwhelmed by life problems, it is often difficult to see a way of addressing these difficulties in a satisfactory way. It can feel impossible to even know where to start. Using a problem-solving approach means stepping back from the problem and considering what solutions exist. A step-by-step approach is taken to identify the problem then consider the potential solutions and the steps required to overcome the problem.

Your current view of problems. How do you currently view stressful problems and your ability to cope with them? If you have a positive attitude towards stressful life problems and your ability to cope with them, then you are more likely to actively try to cope with a problem rather than avoid it. If, on the other hand, you tend to view life problems as a major threat, see yourself as being unable to cope with them and get overwhelmed by negative emotions, then you are likely to do your best to avoid problems.

What is your problem-solving style? This refers to what we do when we are trying to cope with a life problem. There are three main types of coping style:

1. The quick fix style, which might mean that the problem is not dealt with completely.

2. The avoidant style, in which you put off dealing with the problem and might even pretend it doesn't exist or let other people deal with it instead.

3. The rational style, which means that you identify the problem, look for solutions, decide the best way to deal with it, put
that into action and review how it has gone.

Which one fits you best? No prizes for guessing which one is
the most helpful way of dealing with problems!

Stages of problem-solving

1. Identify your problem precisely. The good news is that
you have already done something similar to this if you wrote
a problem statement earlier. In order to begin problem-solving, you could start with your problem statement or you may
wish to focus on something specific in a bit more detail, such
as, 'I'm exhausted every night.' Another example of a specific
problem is: 'I engage in comfort snacking most days, which
plays havoc with my blood glucose.'

2. Write down as many possible solutions as you can. Try
to be as creative as possible when you come to writing down
possible solutions. The idea is not to come up with purely
practical, sensible solutions but to think of all the possibilities,
no matter how outlandish. You can pass judgement on them
later. For now, thinking outside the box is going to help you
to start to think differently about situations that have been
troubling you.

3. Think through the pros and cons for each solution. This
is where you go through the possible solutions you have just
come up with and think about the pros and cons of each one.

To help you begin, rule out any that are immoral, illegal or impractical! You should be left with a few practical possibilities which, if implemented, will improve your life.

4. Select the best possible solution. When considering which potential solution to try out, consider how each option could help you solve your problem. Think about the short- and long-term benefits of each, the time and effort each solution will require and the consequences for you and those around you of choosing that solution.

5. Plan how to carry out the solution. By now you have come up with a potential solution. It is worth thinking about how you will carry out your solution in some detail. Are there any resources you will need? What needs to happen to enable you to try the solution? What particular steps will need to be undertaken?

6. Put the plan into action. Go for it!

7. Review what happens. Once you have carried out your solution, it is now time to evaluate what happened. Did it go better or worse than expected? Take time to record your mood and whatever else you are recording (perhaps anxiety), and see if there have been any changes. If there have been changes, what do you think may have caused them? If there haven't been any positive changes, take a moment to reflect on this, too.

What have you learned from your attempt to problem-solve? What will you take from the experience for the future?

Many people say that they problem-solve in their head rather than writing things down or talking about them. The trouble with this approach is that very often the minds of people who are experiencing problems such as diabetes distress or depression are full of negative thoughts and images, and worries and anxieties. Writing things down can help us to see things from a different point of view and more clearly, so it is worth making a note of your thoughts and ideas as you go through the steps above. You can use the form in the Appendix 3: Resources (for Chapter 10) to do this but first let's see how Nandita went about problem-solving.

Nandita's completed problem-solving steps

Nandita was diagnosed with T2D ten years ago. She takes metformin twice a day and a single injection of long-acting insulin at night. Nandita has struggled with a combination of low mood and anxiety, and feels resentful of her T2D and the restrictions on her life. She retired early from teaching as she was finding it difficult to run her music lessons due to neuropathy (loss of feeling in her hands and feet). She occasionally forgets to take her medication, which she is reluctant to take anyway. But when she doesn't take it she worries. She injects her insulin but hardly ever checks her morning blood glucose, which she knows she should do. She feels guilty for snacking frequently on sweet biscuits.

Table 10.6: Nandita's problem-solving steps

Step 1. Identify your problem precisely I struggle to remember to take my metformin every day.
Step 2. Write down as many possible solutions as you can Don't bother taking it at all. Put a tablet on every surface in every room so there is always one around to remind me. Put them by the kettle so I am reminded to take one every morning. Put them by the bathroom sink so I remember to take one before bed every night. Take a double dose on the days I realise I missed them the day before. Set an alarm on my phone for the same time every day. Ask husband to remind me. Put a note on the fridge. Put a note on the biscuit tin. Just take them when I remember.
Step 3. Think through the pros and cons of each solution.

Solution 1. Don't bother taking it at all.

Pros	Cons
I don't need to worry about a missed dose. It will be like it was before – no tablets!	The doctor said they would help. I risk becoming more ill.

Solution 2. Put a tablet on every surface in every room so there is always one around to remind me.

Pros	Cons
I would be sure to see them somewhere!	I might take more than one by mistake.

Solution 3. Put them by the kettle so I am reminded to take the morning dose.

Pros	Cons
I would see them when I go for my morning coffee.	I need to take it with my evening meal too and don't have a hot drink then so may not notice it.

Solution 4. Put some by the bathroom sink so I remember to take the one before bed every night.

Pros	Cons
I would see them in the morning and before bed.	Bedtime is not the time to take metformin.

Solution 5. Take extra doses on the days I realise I missed them the day before.

Pros	Cons
It might top up my levels?	My diabetes nurse advised against this.

Solution 6. Set an alarm on my phone for the same time every day.

Pros	Cons
I could set my alarm for mealtimes, after all I hardly ever vary the time I eat.	Can't think of any.

Solution 7. Ask husband to remind me.

Pros	Cons
He would feel like he was helping me, which he would like.	He might forget. Unfair to rely on him to do that. Stops me taking responsibility for self-management.

Solution 8. Put a note on the fridge.	
Pros	Cons
I walk past the fridge a lot.	It might trigger me to open the fridge door. I usually go into the fridge when prepping and snack!

Solution 9. Put a note on the biscuit tin.	
Pros	Cons
I would see it when I go in the cupboard.	It could trigger me to want a biscuit. I would need to put the tin on the worktop rather than in the cupboard so would be triggered a lot.

Solution 10. Just take them when I remember.	
Pros	Cons
I might feel more relaxed about it.	I am likely to make myself more ill.

Step 4. Select the best possible solution

Solution 6 seems to be the best solution and is easy to implement.

Step 5. Plan how to carry out the solution

To make sure I do this, I need to set my phone alarm for the same time every day and put it on snooze until I take it.

Step 6. Put the plan into action

Step 7. Review what happens

It went better than expected! I've been doing it for one week and have taken metformin around breakfast and dinner time every day. I don't particularly like taking it but I am getting used to it and it is less on my mind throughout the day, which means I am worrying less, which feels better. Success!

Could a problem-solving strategy be helpful for you? If so, why not give it a go? Try to think of a problem that is affecting you and take your time to go through the problem-solving steps. It could be any problem, not just around your T2D. Allow yourself time to think of outlandish solutions, sometimes the free thinking can enable you to come up with great solutions that you would otherwise not have thought of. Don't worry if it takes a while to do, coming up with a great solution to an ongoing problem is generally worth the effort. Like most things, the more you do it, the quicker you get. When something works well, we feel more motivated to keep going – and try the approach on other problems.

In this chapter, we have looked at how mental health can be affected by a T2D diagnosis. You will have learned how to come up with a problem statement which captures your current difficulties and how to set realistic and measurable goals. We have described how to use behavioural activation and problem-solving, and hopefully you will have had a chance to give one or both a go. We hope this chapter has helped you to start putting together a tool bag of strategies that you can use when needed. Like anything new, these strategies all take practice, so don't be disheartened if you need to give a particular technique a few goes before you get the hang of it. If you have ongoing difficulties with adjusting to your diagnosis of T2D or think you are clinically depressed then please talk to your diabetes healthcare team and/or doctor, who can offer additional advice and support.

Key points from Chapter 10

- A T2D diagnosis can affect mental health.

- Poor mental health can affect T2D.

- Diabetes distress describes the negative emotional response that people have to living with T2D.

- Problem statements are a great way of starting to get to grips with the problem.

- SMART goals are a good way to work towards positive change.

- Behavioural activation is an outside-in approach to when your mood is a barrier to looking after yourself.

- Problem-solving is a straightforward and effective way of finding solutions to everyday life problems.

Looking after your psychological wellbeing: it's the thought that counts

FAS_T_ – dealing with tension, stress, low mood and anxiety part 2

In this chapter, we will continue our focus on the psychological aspect of T2D and present some more useful CBT strategies to add to your wellbeing tool bag to draw on if and when you need them. Specifically, we are going to look at ways to tackle the following:

1. Avoiding uncomfortable thoughts, feelings and physical sensations.

2. Heightened self-focus so that you notice things about yourself more.

3. Ruminating, or going over and over things – worrying much of the time.

Tackling avoidance of uncomfortable thoughts, feelings and physical sensations

Receiving a diagnosis of T2D is hard so it is no wonder that some people try to stop themselves from experiencing unpleasant responses to it.

You might avoid uncomfortable thoughts (including images), feelings or physical sensations in one of two ways: first, by denying that you really have a problem or that T2D might have any long-term consequences; alternatively, you might hide your emotions about it from others so that friends and family are unaware of the distress you are experiencing. Denial and not showing emotions to others are ways of coping with the distress of T2D. This is understandable but not helpful in the long-term.

If you do use one of these coping strategies, you might not see yourself as experiencing T2D distress and those around you would probably agree as you might be showing no outward signs of distress. Indeed, by engaging in denial or hiding your emotions, you might even keep your mood stable – simply by not actually facing up to T2D.

Distraction from the upsetting reality of T2D might appeal, at least in the short-term, but by definition will then prevent you from addressing any T2D-related problem – a very obvious downside. A diagnosis of T2D requires action, and emotional avoidance can be quite a burden, not to mention the potential consequences. Don't just take our word for it. Let's look at a couple of examples.

Denial example. Nandita's T2D has progressed to the point where she needs to take insulin as well as tablets, but she is in denial of the negative consequences of not taking her metformin medication. When faced with information from her healthcare team or images of the potential consequences of not adhering to treatment, Nandita uses distraction to focus her attention away from the problem. Outwardly, Nandita does not appear to be experiencing diabetes distress. She seems emotionally OK even when faced with upsetting T2D-related information.

Suppression example. Benjamin suppresses his emotions about his T2D. Inwardly, he is terrified about it and worries constantly about what the future may hold, but does not express any of these feelings to the people around him. He appears cheerful and bright, like nothing has changed. Friends and family think he is coping amazingly well and they have stopped asking him about it as he makes it clear that it is not a topic for conversation – he is fine! The people close to Benjamin certainly would not think that he is experiencing diabetes distress.

Of course, both Nandita and Benjamin are experiencing distress. Does this affect you? If so, here are some ideas on what you can do about it.

Writing down emotions

What we know is that holding back emotions is stressful and can take its toll – it's exhausting! It can be difficult for some people to confide in others, but writing down your feelings can be easier and many people find it helps. It means setting aside space and time to put pen to paper or fingers to keyboard to write about your experience of T2D and how it makes you feel. It can be useful to do this more than once, perhaps on three or four consecutive days. Doing this alone can help get those emotions out and allow you to begin processing them. Sometimes writing down emotions such as anger, anxiety or low mood can highlight thoughts and beliefs about T2D and its treatment that might well be wrong, and a rethink may be needed! Writing down your emotions can also help identify unhelpful problem-solving styles that you can do something about, which has the bonus of helping you become an effective T2D self-manager.

Of course, some of the beliefs and emotions you write down could well be understandable yet still need action. When this is the case, it can be helpful to reflect on the pros and cons of your current coping styles and any longer-term consequences to help you reach a place of acceptance. We will come on to this shortly. Before we do that, this is a good time to look at your thoughts and beliefs around illness and treatment. Here are some **common thoughts and beliefs about T2D**. Make a note of the ones that apply to you and any others that you experience that are not included here.

- 'I cannot do anything to control my T2D'

- 'T2D has taken over my life'

- 'My life is ruined'

- 'Why me?'

- 'Nothing can ever be as good again'

- 'I've let everyone down'

- 'Treatment won't help'

Writing about emotions can be difficult and you may find it helpful to talk to someone first if you think you would like to try this exercise.

Using a cost–benefit analysis

We know that you can naturally want to avoid experiencing unpleasant responses to a T2D diagnosis. However, denying or distracting yourself from the upsetting reality of T2D has a downside to it. Avoiding facing up to T2D also can mean avoiding addressing the T2D itself, and this is when doing a cost–benefit analysis can be helpful (think of pros and cons if that helps).

A cost–benefit analysis is a way of analysing which decisions to make and which not to. The cost–benefit analysis allows you to sum up the potential rewards expected from given actions after subtracting the costs associated with them. It often works best if you give each action a score out of 100 as to how important it is to you, with 0 being not important at all and 100 being of maximum importance. Let's look at a cost–benefit analysis that Nandita did of her denial strategies.

Table 11.1: Nandita – the costs and benefits of denying that I have T2D

Benefits (pros)		Costs (cons)	
Describe	Importance (0–100%)	Describe	Importance (0–100%)
I don't get upset.	90	When I do think about it I get very anxious.	90
I can carry on as normal.	90	I risk long-term problems if I don't act.	100
I don't need to go to hospital appointments.	60	I risk dying sooner than I should.	100
No boring conversations about tests.	80	Better blood glucose would make me feel more energetic – now.	100
My family are not affected by my changing things.	80	If I die early I will miss watching the grandkids grow up.	100
		I will have given up the opportunity to get control over my diabetes, or the chance of putting it into remission.	100
	400		590

Totals 400 and 590 = a cost of 190.

Nandita did this after reading about self-management of T2D, having been previously unaware of the possibility of putting T2D into remission or that she might just feel better in herself *right now* if her blood glucose was better controlled.

As you can see from this cost–benefit analysis, Nandita has identified a number of perceived benefits of getting on with life while denying she has T2D. The rating is high. However, the costs are even higher, and when reading it all through Nandita is able to see that the short-term benefits are outweighed by the costs – a mixture of 'here and now' and longer-term consequences. In addition, she is unable to shut out *all* thoughts about her T2D, including missing hospital appointments, which still keeps her feeling upset, so she never actually experiences the full rewards of her denial strategy. Her family want to support her but by carrying on as normal she is not able to embrace that help and use it to her advantage.

If this problem applies to you, this is a good time to try doing your own cost–benefit analysis. It tends to work best if you write it down and ensure you set time aside to give it some serious thought. We recommend you only do this if you have read the previous sections of the book.

Working on thoughts

In diabetes distress and depression, people can be prone to certain ways of thinking, and some common thinking errors. A particularly common thinking error is when a person focuses on the negative and discounts the positive sides of things. For example, a person might focus on the negative impact of T2D and discount everything else positive in their life. Cognitive techniques can help a person to come up with a more balanced view of their T2D by acknowledging that aspects of T2D life can be a negative experience – such as restricted eating or socialising – but counterbalancing this with aspects of life it doesn't affect, such as reading or spending time with grandchildren. This is not the same as positive thinking – that would involve just focusing on the good stuff. What we are looking for is a balance of acknowledging the negative whilst not ignoring the positive.

It's possible sometimes that negative thoughts come from beliefs that can be challenged – a new eating approach might be just different rather than restricted. It might even be an adventure! Table 11.2 shows how our thoughts (our interpretation of an event) affect our emotions, physical feelings and behaviour.

11.2 Linking behaviours to thoughts, emotions and bodily sensations

Situation	Thought	Emotion	Physical	Behaviour
You are meeting a friend at 6 p.m. It is now 6.30 and your friend is nowhere to be seen.	My friend is never late . . . something awful must have happened . . . he must have been involved in a car crash.	Worry and anxiety	Racing heart, shaking	Call his mobile, home, work, partner and maybe even the police.
	He obviously finds me so dull that he has forgotten about meeting me . . . why would anyone want to meet up with me? I can't blame him . . . I am so forgettable . . . I am such a loser.	Sadness	Sinking feeling in the pit of stomach, tearful	Go home and retreat to bed.
	Well this just shows exactly how selfish he is . . . imagine not even turning up . . . how dare he . . . who the hell does he think he is?	Anger	Tense muscles, flushing	Phone him at home and leave an angry message and block any of his calls.

How awful, everyone is looking at me . . . they think I've been stood up . . . I bet I've gone bright red.	Humiliation and embarrassment	Feeling hot, sweaty, blushing	Look down, try to avoid eye contact, fidget.
Yikes, did we agree this restaurant? I know we talked about another restaurant, which is on the other side of town . . . I bet I'm in the wrong place and he is waiting for me there.	Anxiety	Racing heart, feeling hot	Try to find phone number for other restaurant and call to see if he is there.
I noticed that the traffic was getting pretty heavy when I arrived, I was lucky to have missed it . . . he is probably caught up in it.	Unconcerned	No change	Perhaps browse through the menu to decide what to order when he shows up.

Changing unhelpful thinking patterns

The four symptom areas shown in Table 11.2 (thoughts, emotions, physical sensations and behaviour) all interact with each other within every one of us. Sometimes it is not always obvious which symptoms should go under a particular heading; for example, would you put 'tearfulness' under physical sensations, emotions or behaviour? Would you put 'feeling slowed down' under behaviour or physical sensations? Where would 'feeling on edge' go – under emotions or physical sensations? The answer is that they should go wherever makes most sense to you.

What is important is being able to tell the difference between thoughts and emotions. This can be confusing because we often talk about thoughts as though they are emotions. For example, 'I feel like he is annoyed with me' is not an emotion despite the words 'I feel'. This is a thought because there is no 'he is annoyed with me' emotion. A more accurate representation of what the person might be trying to say would be something like, 'I think he is really angry with me and it is making me feel anxious.' In this sentence, anxiety is an emotion that is being expressed in a thought. It is very common for us to talk about our feelings when we are talking about our thoughts (e.g. 'I feel he doesn't like me', 'I feel like I'll get into big trouble for this'). Emotions tend to be expressed in just one word, like angry, anxious, sad, embarrassed, guilty, frightened, worried, upset and so on. This is important to remember when we come on to thought diaries later.

Cognitive behavioural therapy is based on the idea that the

way we make sense of events affects how we feel and what we do. It is not the event itself that makes us feel a certain way, otherwise everyone would react in exactly the same way to a given situation – and we know that is not the case. You will be able to think of lots of examples of when one of your family or friends has viewed something completely differently to you. Even being diagnosed with T2D will not result in the same response from everyone. So why is this? In CBT, we believe the range of different reactions triggered in people by a particular situation is a result of the range of different thoughts or interpretations that the given situation triggers in those people. The example in Table 11.2 shows how one situation can be interpreted in a number of different ways.

The problem is that most of us have a tendency to just accept our thoughts as true and leave them unchecked. If we were right all of the time then that would be fine, but as we can see from the restaurant example in Table 11.2, this is unlikely to be the case. Many of us treat our thoughts like they are facts (for example, 'I know that she hates me'). However, just because we *believe* a given thought, it does not make it a fact. If John thinks his favourite book is the best book in the world, it does not mean that this book is actually the best, and Pam may disagree! In just the same way, if you think you are a failure, it does not mean that you *are* a failure.

Unpleasant and upsetting thoughts tend to be automatic; they just pop into mind, unlike purposeful thoughts, which occur when we consciously turn our minds to something. Automatic thoughts can be positive, negative or neutral. A positive automatic thought might be, 'I love my new shirt', triggered by passing a mirror. A neutral automatic thought might be, 'Ah, I need to pick up some coffee', triggered by walking past the coffee aisle in a supermarket. Negative automatic thoughts tend to be rapid and brief, and the content harsh and usually highly convincing (for example, 'I'm such a failure for getting T2D'). Negative automatic thoughts generally lead to equally negative emotions.

Going back to Figure 10.1 on page 293, the reason we placed 'emotion' at the top is because we are often most aware of the feelings that the situation produces but it is actually the thought that has triggered the emotion. Moreover, how strongly we feel the emotion will be determined by how strongly we believe the thought, which will also impact our physical sensations and what we do (our behaviour). Think back to the example in Table 11.2.

In summary, our reactions following an event are most likely to be:

Event → Thought/interpretation →
Reactions (emotions, bodily sensations and behaviours)

Instead of:

Event → Reactions

When we realise that the problems we're experiencing are not caused directly by events but rather by our *interpretation* of those events, it makes sense to try to tackle some of those interpretations. To help you do this, it's worth being aware of some patterns of thinking that are common and can be particularly troublesome for people experiencing emotional problems. These are usually referred to as 'thinking errors'. We have listed some of the key thinking errors in Table 11.3, along with examples of how they work in the lives of the people with T2D.

Table 11.3: Thinking errors

Thinking error	Description	Example
'All or nothing' or 'black and white' thinking	You do not do things by halves – there is no middle ground or shades of grey. People are either successful or a failure; they either like you or hate you; you are either right or wrong.	'I ate three cookies with a cup of tea. I am completely useless.'
Overgeneralising	You take one specific event and apply it to lots of others in your life; this includes a negative evaluation of yourself.	Your doctor told you that you need to lose weight. 'Everyone thinks I'm fat.'
Minimising and maximising	You blow things out of proportion, making mountains out of molehills; you underplay and undervalue your strengths but emphasise your weaknesses.	Being worried about an imminent check-up. 'Getting a bad test result proves just how inadequate I am', although getting a good one doesn't really mean anything.

Fortune-telling	You predict that things will turn out badly, no matter what you say or do.	Concluding that there is no point in taking diabetes medication every day as your T2D is going to get worse anyway.
Emotional reasoning	You base your judgement of the situation on how you are feeling. You *feel* anxious so you *think* there must be danger.	Feeling guilty after having a glass of wine and nibbles after a tough day at work and concluding 'I'm a waste of space', rather than seeing yourself as others would – as someone who is doing incredibly well in very difficult circumstances.
Selective abstracting	You focus on one negative aspect of an event rather than taking all aspects into account.	After having a good week going for walks every day, on the last day you didn't go out and sat watching TV most of the day. Rather than congratulating yourself for increasing your activity over the week you are preoccupied by the day you didn't go for a walk, which makes you feel anxious and upset.

Discounting the positive	You discount positive things about yourself.	Having been praised by the diabetes nurse for improving your HbA1c after a lot of effort you dismiss the compliment because 'anyone could have done that'.
Personalising	When something goes wrong, you blame yourself. The same is not true when things go right.	After having made a mushroom risotto for friends, you discover during the meal that one of your friends does not like mushrooms. You blame yourself for not remembering this and discount all the times you made meals that all your friends enjoyed.
Mind-reading	You think you know what others are thinking. This is very common and usually involves believing they are thinking something bad about you.	'I texted Andrew two days ago to see if he wanted to meet up but have not heard back. He thinks I'm such bad company now that I have T2D.'

Why are these thinking patterns important? How we think affects how we feel and behave, as well as what happens in our body. Our thoughts, emotions, bodily sensations and behaviour are all interconnected. Can you take a compliment?

No? Imagine that someone says, 'You're looking good today.' If you think, 'They are only saying that, they don't really mean it' (thinking error: 'discounting the positive'/'mind reading'), then you are likely to continue to feel low. If, on the other hand, you can say 'Thank you', and believe that you are truly looking well, then such a compliment is likely to improve your mood.

In general, if you are prone to thinking the worst, changing this aspect of your thinking is going to be important in helping you to reduce your heightened emotion. If you tend to discount the positive aspects of yourself, changing that thinking error should improve how you feel about yourself.

EXERCISE

Identifying my thinking errors

Think back to a recent event that triggered feelings of anxiety, low mood, anger or stress in general. Can you identify your thoughts, then any thinking errors? Either use the form in Appendix 3: Resources (for Chapter 11) or simply make a note of the event, your feelings, thoughts and possible thinking errors.

Identifying interpretations

What we know so far is that our feelings, thoughts and behaviours are closely related. Now we'll look in more depth at the kinds of thoughts that occur automatically in various

situations. In particular, we will focus on the negative interpretations of events that arise automatically and that lead us to
experience a negative emotion.

Thought diaries. Let's look at examples of automatic thinking
with Nandita's, Colin's and Benjamin's thought diaries.

Table 11.4: Nandita's thought diary

Date	Situation	Emotion	Thought
Include day of week and time of day where relevant	Where were you? What were you doing? Who were you with?	**Rate intensity 0–100 per cent**	What was going through your head just as you started to feel the emotion? List all thoughts and images. **Rate belief 0–100 per cent and circle the most upsetting thought**
Fri 6th	Sitting watching TV but unable to concentrate. Thoughts about how bleak my future is with T2D keep on coming to mind.	Sad 100%	I should have realised that something wasn't right before my hands started tingling (80%) I'll never feel truly happy again (100%)

Table 11.5: Colin's thought diary

Date	Situation	Emotion	Thought
Include day of week and time of day where relevant	Where were you? What were you doing? Who were you with?	**Rate intensity 0–100 per cent**	What was going through your head just as you started to feel the emotion? List all thoughts and images. **Rate belief 0–100 per cent and circle the most upsetting thought**
Tues 14th	Appointment card arrives for first diabetes appointment.	Miserable 100%	What's the point in going to the appointment? I can't take all this in (90%) I'm ready for the scrapheap (100%)

You may have noticed that Colin included a question in his thought column, but that it remained unrated. That is because it is very difficult to rate your belief in a question. If you do have a question in mind, it's best to turn it into a statement. Your rating will then indicate how much of a question mark there is over that statement. For example, 'What's the point in going to the appointment?' could be changed to, 'There is no point in going to the appointment' and Colin could rate how much he believes this statement. The higher he rates it, the more certain he feels about it.

Table 11.6: Benjamin's thought diary

Date	Situation	Emotion	Thought
Include day of week and time of day where relevant	Where were you? What were you doing? Who were you with?	**Rate intensity 0–100 per cent**	What was going through your head just as you started to feel the emotion? List all thoughts and images. **Rate belief 0–100 per cent and circle the most upsetting thought**
Mon 5th, 8:30 a.m.	Realised this morning that I forgot to take my medication last night.	Worried 70% Upset 90%	This is really bad for my T2D (70%) I cannot get to grips with this life change (90%) I never get anything right (95%)

Note that all the emotions are described in one word (i.e. sad, miserable, worried, upset) and that it is possible to experience more than one emotion at a time. When you make your own thought diary, remember that the emotion should make sense in relation to the thought you are recording. For example, let's say you found yourself in a large department store and rated your anxiety at 70 per cent. Your emotion isn't linked to your thought that 'this place is enormous', but instead to the thought that 'I'm going to panic and not be able to find my way out of here.' Look back over the examples in Tables 11.4–11.6 and think whether you would feel the same as Nandita, Colin and Benjamin if you believed their thoughts as much as they did. Would you feel differently, and if so in what way? Why do you think you would feel differently? The answer to this question is likely to be that you would interpret the situation in a different way from the person in the example.

EXERCISE

Your Thought Diary

Now it's time to try this exercise for yourself. You can use the thought diary template in Appendix 3: Resources (for Chapter 11).

1. First, think back to a recent upsetting event and write down the answers to the following questions:

- When was it? Put the date in the first column.

- What was the event or situation? Where were you? What were you doing? Who were you with? Write this down in the second column.

- What was the emotion you experienced (e.g. anger, sadness, anxiety)? Remember, this is likely to just be one word. Write this in the third column.

- What went through your mind at the time (e.g. 'Nobody understands')? Remember that it is best to turn any questions into statements. Add this to the fourth column.

2. Now take a moment to rate the intensity of the emotion you felt at the time using a percentage scale where 0 is not at all, 100 per cent is extremely high intensity and 50 per cent is moderate. Feel free to be as specific as you want with the number you select.

3. Once you've done that, take another moment to rate how much you believed the thought that went through your mind at the time. If there were lots of thoughts (and very often many negative thoughts come rushing into our minds at times like this), then circle the one that is most upsetting.

Now you have had a go at completing the four-column thought diary, the next step is to use the diary over the next week. This time, complete the diary *as and when* strong feelings occur. There are a couple of good reasons for this. First, if you write things down when the events are fresh in your mind, the information you record about your thoughts and possible thinking errors is more likely to be accurate. Second, writing things down is a way of distancing yourself from your thoughts. It will help you to think more objectively about your thoughts and the situation and thus make it easier to break any negative thinking habits. Find a four-column thought diary in Appendix 3: Resources (for Chapter 11).

Evaluating interpretations

It is a good idea to get some practice at identifying and recording your thinking in various situations you find upsetting, as well as recording your thinking errors before moving on to evaluating your thoughts. Evaluating thoughts can be a powerful strategy in dealing with difficult emotions.

We'll now look in depth at how to change your thinking by identifying your thinking errors. In addition, you will learn to check whether there is any information you can use to challenge the interpretation of events that causes you distress, and to help you arrive at an alternative perspective. We call this 'evaluating thoughts' because weighing up the evidence for and against a given thought helps you judge whether it's valid or not. We will go through this process now with another example from Benjamin.

Table 11.7: Benjamin's 9-column Thought Diary

Date Include day of week and time of day where relevant	Situation	Emotion Rate intensity 0–100%	Thought Rate belief 0–100% and circle the most upsetting thought	Evidence for the most upsetting thought	Evidence against the most upsetting thought	Alternative thought and rate belief in it	Re-rate belief in upsetting thought and intensity of emotion	What to do next
Mon 5th	At work at a colleague's leaving event. Someone was handing out slices of cake and asked if I was 'allowed' a bit given I had T2D.	Upset 100%	I am being treated differently because of my T2D (100%) Everyone is looking at me and feeling sorry for me (80%) Yet again T2D ruins my day (100%)	I either eat the cake and feel guilty or don't have it and feel like I am missing out. It is only me that has T2D.	This is all or nothing thinking. I can still join in without having cake. I can still say goodbye to my colleague and have a laugh without eating cake.	Although I would enjoy the cake, I can still do the rest of the things that everyone else is doing to celebrate with my colleague getting a new job so T2D has not ruined my day. The reality is that I can enjoy the event without the cake! (70%)	Belief in thought 60% Upset 50%	Try to embrace the moment and the elements of a situation I can enjoy without focusing on one thing that I cannot do.

EXERCISE

Your nine-column thought diary

Think about the past few days, and try to select examples of when you became distressed, whether that be angry, anxious, depressed or you felt low about yourself. Can you identify any of your own thinking errors?

Step 1. Choose an example of something that happened that caused you some distress. Try not to choose the most distressing event or situation, as it could be overwhelming and difficult to use the strategy right away (you can do that once you get the hang of it). Identify the main emotion experienced in the situation and rate its intensity (0–100%). Next, identify the thoughts you had, rate how much you believed them, and circle the most upsetting thought. Can you spot a thinking error? Use the nine-column thought diary in Appendix 3: Resources (for Chapter 11) to help you.

Step 2. Now consider the evidence that exists for the most upsetting thought being true. If you find this tricky, ask yourself the following questions:

- What is the evidence you have for the upsetting thought?

- What makes you come to that conclusion?

- You believe the thought ___ %. What is it that makes you believe it so strongly?

Write the answers to these questions in the 'Evidence for the most upsetting thought' column. Be careful only to use factual evidence rather than another negative thought. For instance, 'Everybody can see I'm anxious' is likely to be another negative thought unless you have been told by every single person where you are that you appear anxious. Similarly, 'Something always goes wrong' is also likely to be another negative thought (an overgeneralisation) because it is most unlikely that absolutely everything goes wrong. 'I've never achieved anything' is also definitely not true and another overgeneralisation. Facts, on the other hand, are things that are indisputable. 'I felt upset when I forgot to take my medication yesterday' is an example of a fact.

Step 3. Next, think about the evidence against your most upsetting thought. If you're prone to a particular thinking error, you can include that here. To help you gather evidence against your most upsetting thought, ask yourself the following questions:

- Does this thought fall into the category of a thinking error? If so, which one?

- What evidence is there that does not support this thought?

- If you rated your belief in the thought as under 100 per cent, it shows an element of doubt. What is that doubt?

- Are there any things that you might be ignoring because you think they are not important, even though they would actually work against this thought?

- What happened last time you were in a situation like this?

- What experiences have you had that would indicate that this thought is not necessarily true?

- Is there another way of looking at this situation?

- What is the worst thing that could happen even if this thought is true?

- If the thought is true, will it still matter in five years' time?

- How might someone else think in this situation?

- If you were not experiencing low mood/depression/distress/anxiety, would you believe this thought?

- What would you say to a friend or family member if they were in the same situation?

Step 4. You now need to think of an alternative explanation for the event and rate your belief in it. Thinking of an alternative thought is not always easy to do, sometimes a friend or family member is able to help with this, but it is still good to be able to do it on your own. What is most important here is that the alternative thought is believable to you. CBT is not about groundless positive thinking but about being realistic. It is absolutely critical that the alternative thought is credible and consistent with what is going on in your life right now.

The key question you need to consider is: taking into account the evidence for and against the thought, can you come up with a more realistic and helpful alternative thought?

Step 5. Having come up with a more realistic alternative thought, re-rate your belief in the upsetting thought and also the intensity of the emotion associated with the thought. Have they changed?

If they have gone down, that's great. You now have a proven method of evaluating the thoughts that are causing you emotional distress. If they have not changed for the better, that is important too. Why do you think that is? Where did you get stuck? Was it that the original thought was too intense and it was just not possible to gather the evidence to help you think in a different way? If this is the case, practise the technique with a less intense thought then build up to your most intense and difficult thoughts. Don't be disheartened. After all, you've probably thought and felt this way for a while. Like trying a new sport or learning to play the piano – thinking in a different way is bound to take time and practice!

What if your negative thought is actually true? It is important to remember that our automatic thoughts are not *always* wrong! They can be true, false or partly true. For example, the thoughts 'I have a life-changing health condition' or 'My blood glucose is not under control' might be true. If this is the case, problem-solving can be a better approach to take (see Chapter 10).

Step 6. The final step is all about what you *do* in the given situation. This is a vitally important stage. If you do not behave any differently, then evaluating your thoughts will have less of an impact on your mood. If, however, you can combine thinking differently with *behaving* differently, then you are on the right path to recovery.

Continue to practise evaluating your interpretations. Gathering evidence to evaluate your interpretations of events and help reduce your distressing emotions is a fundamental part of effective CBT. For this reason, we recommend you spend the next week or so practising this skill. At the end of each day, take a few moments to reflect on how things are going with your evaluations. What is going well and what requires more effort or some help? If you are getting stuck, use problem-solving to help you. You are likely to find thought evaluation most helpful if you can do it at the time of the event or as close to the time as possible. It is also important that you write things down rather than just doing the exercises in your head; that way you become much more aware of the steps in the process and can go back to previous diaries when needed.

Tackling heightened self-focus

When you are told that you have a potentially serious long-term condition, it can be difficult not to attribute any bodily sensation to that condition, whether that's a realistic appraisal of it or not. If we overly scan our bodies we can always find things to occupy our thoughts, and even normal body sensations can become symptoms when we are being over-vigilant.

Learning about T2D is one way to be able to understand whether sensations might be symptoms and whether either matter or not. Most people with T2D, most of the time, have no symptoms other than tiredness. We've covered the symptoms of changes in blood glucose, and if you are able to self-monitor glucose you will quickly be able to tell whether sensations are linked to that. If self-monitoring is not an option, then discuss persistent or recurrent symptoms with your healthcare practitioner before jumping to a conclusion. It is well worth learning the difference between a sensation and a symptom – try this exercise.

EXERCISE

Sensation awareness

For the next two or three minutes focus your attention on your left hand. Do not move it, just concentrate on any sensations you experience. You can close your eyes to help you concentrate or you may want to look at your hand during the exercise. When the time has elapsed, answer the following questions:

1. Did you experience any of the following symptoms: heaviness, warmth, tingling, shakiness, other sensation, or nothing?

2. Were you aware of any of the sensations prior to the exercise?

If you experienced any sensations during this exercise that you had not noticed before, this highlights what's called selective attention. If you experienced no sensations, try the exercise again but for a little longer this time. Try focusing on another part of your body as well (e.g. your feet, eyes) and see what happens.

What does it mean? This experiment demonstrates how sensations that you were not aware of previously can become obvious or heightened when you focus attention on them. So although there is a definite need to self-monitor and be self-aware, there is a balance to be struck.

A changed view of self. Another unhelpful focus of attention can be if the way you see yourself (with T2D) does not fit with how you would like to see yourself. There has been a change! We said earlier that you *could* focus on the negative impacts of T2D to the detriment of anything positive in your life. Having T2D is difficult, we know that, but it does not mean that your life is ruined. Lots of the positives that were in your life before are still there whether that be family, friends, work or hobbies, etc. Learning how to identify when you are engaging in this 'discounting of the positives' of life can be really helpful.

Try using a thought diary – see earlier in this chapter and Appendix 3: Resources (for Chapter 11) – to work through evaluating unhelpful or upsetting thoughts which can otherwise generate negative emotions and impair the way you view yourself. You will have evidence supporting your negative thoughts of course, such as, 'It's much harder now to eat out with friends', but this can be counterbalanced with those parts of life it does not impact, such as gardening or going to the sports centre or cinema, and just *being* with friends. Give a thought diary a try, as we described earlier.

Tackling rumination and worry

Rumination – we all do it! The key difference as to whether it is useful or not is whether these thoughts lead to problem-solving (helpful) or brooding (unhelpful). Persistent negative thinking is not uncommon when we are in distress and can often include a focus on loss and/or worries about the future. Rumination on a diagnosis of T2D and its implications is natural and reflects the importance of your concerns about real-life difficulties. When we are in distress, rumination can be automatic, frequent and hard to control.

Do you dwell on thoughts such as 'Why me?' Do you think over and over about what you did to deserve being diagnosed with T2D? Do you find that you spend long periods worrying about what the future holds? Ruminating and worrying means that you really *want* to problem-solve the thing you are think-ing about, but ruminating itself can actually *prevent* you from doing so. For instance, Nandita ruminates about the unfair-ness of developing T2D, frequently thinking: 'Why did I get a diagnosis of T2D when no one else in my family has it?', 'T2D has ruined my life', 'My future is bleak.' This rumination stops Nandita from taking action as she is stuck in this particular thinking loop.

Rumination and worry tend to make us feel worse and do nothing to motivate us to do anything about them; they make us mull over things rather than moving us to action. Helpful thinking, by contrast, leads to actions and solutions. Nandita's thoughts would get anyone down if they were churning around in their mind for long periods. In addition, science tells us that rumination can increase our risk of becoming depressed and can help keep depression going.

EXERCISE

Rumination

Imagine that your computer/laptop suddenly switches off without warning. It is helpful to take a bit of time to think of why it might have done that and to consider possible reasons for the problem; is it plugged into the wall, has the plug fused, does it have a virus? Thinking this through will help you to solve the problem and to move to action such as plugging it into the wall and trying to switch it on! Simply thinking about it won't solve the problem. Also, just trying an action without thinking through the problem may not solve it (repeatedly clicking the 'on' button). What this shows is that balance is key. Asking 'Why me?' can leave you stuck. Asking 'Why is the laptop not working?' and 'How do I fix it?' helps you focus on addressing the problem. Likewise, 'Why me?' when it comes to a T2D diagnosis does not help. 'What can I do to fix it?' calls you to action. 'How can I fix it?' helps you to focus on the current problem and do something about it, while 'Why me?' leads to a self-focus and can progress to unhelpful feelings of self-blame.

Interestingly, Cassie experienced both reactions when she was diagnosed with T2D – with 'How can I fix it?' being dominant – which led to her action-orientated response to having T2D.

Although most of us do ruminate from time to time, it becomes unhelpful when it is a habit and an automatic response to upsetting thoughts. Habits are learned, therefore with practice they can be unlearned, which is good news when it comes to rumination. You are likely to have broken unhelpful habits before in your life. For example, maybe you smoked or bit your nails. The way to change a habit is to become aware of what triggers it and then do something more helpful instead. It does take practice to change a habit, as you will know. Noticing early warning signs and doing something different helps. Thought evaluation and problem-solving can help, as can changing 'why' questions to 'how' questions. When we are ruminating it can feel almost like we have a running commentary going through our minds.

Perhaps now is a good time to try to pay attention to whether there is a time or place that triggers your rumination. Keep an eye out for early warning signs that you are about to start ruminating, then once you have spotted a pattern, try to do something different. If we see rumination as a bad habit, how have you broken a bad habit before? What helped? When you created a good habit, what helped? The thing with new habits is that they need to be practised repeatedly until they become automatic, so you don't fall back into old ways. It takes practice and you need to be kind to yourself when there are the inevitable lapses. Part of diet failure is often that the 'new way' has not become easy or comfortable enough to replace the 'old way'. Not falling back into old ways is at the heart of the T2D challenge.

Absorbing activities. A useful way of breaking the cycle of rumination is to do something else that is absorbing – something in which you become completely engrossed, taking up all your attention and energy. The concentration and focus involved in losing ourselves makes it very hard to feel low or anxious, or worry. It can be helpful to schedule positive, absorbing activities that make it almost impossible to engage in repetitive thinking, just like the scheduling in behavioural activation in Chapter 10.

What we find absorbing is very individual. It could be something creative, artistic, sporty – pretty much anything where you are completely focused on what you are doing. For instance, learning how to play the guitar, and being absorbed by reading the music and where to put your fingers for different sounds. Ideally, it should be something that connects with your interests and skills but is challenging enough to need your concentration.

Nandita found that once she had engaged in something that she found absorbing (music software on her computer), it gave her a welcome rest from her worries. She was then able to better engage in problem-solving and managing unhelpful thoughts. She examined the benefits of remaining focused on the injustice of her T2D diagnosis relative to focusing on what she could do and achieving her long-term life goals. By doing a cost–benefit analysis, she was able to shift her focus on the aspects of her T2D that were outside her control to factors that she could control, which helped her become a better T2D self-manager using an effective problem-solving style. This shift in focus also provided opportunities for enjoyment and a sense of mastery and accomplishment (think behavioural activation – Chapter 10).

John finds playing the piano absorbing. Pam gets lost in pastel painting. What activities do you find absorbing? You might need to think back a bit if there is nothing that immediately comes to mind. Make a list of a few activities where you have been completely absorbed in what you were doing. The idea is to then engage in one or other of these activities at times when you may be prone to rumination. It can mean having all the equipment you need easily to hand (e.g. art materials) and it takes practice, so don't be too hard on yourself if it takes a few goes before you notice the benefits.

Being kind to yourself

Sometimes worrying thoughts would be seen as valid by almost everyone (e.g. 'I could become very ill'), yet rumination is still not helpful as it does not bring about change. Another strategy that can help is taking a more compassionate stance. For instance, Benjamin experienced episodes of self-blame: 'I brought this on myself' and 'I deserve this.' He could be extremely hard on himself. Do you do this? If so, remember the more caring and nurturing feelings that you have for other people in your life and try to apply them to yourself.

Changing how we talk to ourselves internally can help make us more compassionate. For instance, 'nobody is perfect' is true, and important to remember. Focus on the progress you are making – 'I went for a twenty-minute walk every day this week, I wasn't doing that last week.' Try to highlight what you are doing well. Remind yourself of previous successes – 'I overcame my fear of the dentist' – especially things that show personal strengths such as your determination. Remind yourself that this is a difficult position to be in and that most people would find it hard to make the changes you are making. Also, remind yourself that you can do this, just take one step at a time. The importance of emphasising the positives in your life, around an issue or in a situation, is something that we hear repeatedly in the experiences of people managing diabetes well.

When working through negative thoughts you learned to ask yourself what you might say to someone else in your position. Let's switch it a little and try asking yourself, 'What would I say to myself if I was being kinder and more compassionate towards myself?' Benjamin used this strategy to be less hard on himself when things weren't going well. Might taking a kinder, more compassionate approach to *yourself* be useful? Give it a try! Think of something kind to say to yourself; perhaps you can focus on something you have changed for the better, a personal strength, etc. Remind yourself that nobody is perfect and that we all make mistakes. Remind yourself that most people would find a T2D diagnosis upsetting and difficult to manage at first. Try to break things down into steps to make them more manageable.

In this chapter, we have continued our focus on mental well-being and strategies to use when things are difficult. We have described a number of CBT strategies that have been shown to help emotional distress, including: writing about emotions, learning to analyse the costs and benefits of thoughts and actions, being able to reset thoughts, absorbing activity to help with rumination, and most importantly being kind to oneself. Hopefully, we've provided you with extra skills to include in your tool bag of strategies that you can use when needed. Like those described in Chapter 10, these approaches all need practice, so don't be disheartened if you need to give a particular technique a few goes before you notice the benefits. Please remember, if you have ongoing difficulties with adjusting to your diagnosis of T2D or think you are clinically depressed, talk to your diabetes healthcare team or doctor for help, advice and signposting to other agencies if needed.

Key points from Chapter 11

- Writing down emotions can sometimes be easier than telling others about them, at least at first.

- A cost–benefit analysis allows you to analyse which decisions to make and which not to.

- Our interpretation (thoughts) of an event will affect our emotions, physical symptoms and behaviours.

- Thinking errors are common and can be troublesome – learning how to spot them can help.

- A good way to start looking at your thoughts is to keep a thought diary.

- Learning how to evaluate the accuracy of thoughts rather than letting them go unchecked is a useful skill.

- When diagnosed with T2D, it can be difficult not to attribute any physical sensation to it, whether that's a realistic appraisal of it or not.

- For some people, a diagnosis of T2D can change the way they view themselves.

- A useful way of breaking the cycle of rumination is to do something absorbing.

- Importantly, take a kind, compassionate approach to yourself – remember, nobody is perfect.

Closing summary

Before we begin our summary of key points from the book, we want to share with you a little more of the onward journeys of our case examples. We hope that their personal stories, based on real events, have helped to demonstrate the wide range of T2D experiences. Nearly everyone diagnosed with T2D will experience one or more negative emotions to begin with. However, the impacts of what is undoubtedly a life-changing diagnosis *can* be overcome.

Cassie

Cassie was diagnosed at the age of fifty-six, with the most symptoms and highest HbA1c of our little group. She was determined to learn as much as she could about T2D and to get control of her health. Cassie reversed her T2D and held her remission until we last met up with her. At the age of fifty-nine, she was well, working normally and exercising much more moderately than before she became ill. Her life adjustment was complex but she was adapting to being without T2D, maintaining her remission on a very low-carbohydrate diet. Her social life changed but friendships if anything were strengthened.

She valued being able to say, 'I no longer have type 2 diabetes, and for good measure, I've stopped drinking alcohol.'

Suzanne

Much of Chapter 9 was about Suzanne and her daughter Chloe. Suzanne developed T2D at a time when she was experiencing a number of life stressors. Although not depressed, she experienced diabetes distress. She used techniques from Chapter 11 to successfully tackle her uncomfortable thoughts and feelings about her T2D. We leave her at the age of forty-eight, still in remission from her T2D, eating a low-carbohydrate diet, and having established a new relationship with (less) alcohol. She has resolved to attend 'early warning' regular medical reviews, in case her T2D reappears. More importantly, perhaps, is that these checks include Chloe. Both have come to understand the importance of Chloe's health to *her* own future and any children she might have. They have a weight maintenance pact which is working for them.

Mustafa

Mustafa had been gaining weight and numbers on his blood pressure throughout his forties. When he started working a shift rotation at aged fifty, his weight climbed steeply and T2D surfaced. He successfully navigated Ramadan while on insulin, which further developed the relationship with his doctor, a fellow Muslim. The doctor later engaged in an educational programme on low-carbohydrate eating in T2D, which helped

Mustafa lose weight and improve his T2D. Mustafa was able to stop insulin but stayed with metformin. He had never thought it possible that he would manage without insulin, and hopes T2D remission might be within reach. His employers have allowed him to stop shift working, which not only enabled him to put into practice strategies to improve his sleep but will definitely improve his chance of achieving remission.

Margaret

Margaret initially followed standard dietary advice and cut back on food. She started exercising and attended gym classes with a friend, but then injured her knee, lost her exercise momentum and discipline with her diet. She used a very low-calorie diet to achieve remission of her T2D but struggled to maintain both. She managed to return to gym classes which helped her mood, and she continues on metformin, with her HbA1c reflecting 'excellent' control. She would like to consider other options for T2D remission but is concerned that the higher fat content of a low-carbohydrate diet might harm her health further, despite the lack of evidence of that being the case. Balancing the potential risks of this (very low or nil) compared to the much higher risks of having T2D could help her.

Ted

Ted was diagnosed with T2D at seventy-eight. He had mild symptoms and never really felt unwell. He had reasonable blood pressure and a HbA1c that was typically under 60mmol/mol (< 7.6%) regarded as 'satisfactory'. He had followed a path many choose: minor adjustments to his lifestyle, some medication and regular checks. Ted had a relaxed attitude to life, which was perhaps helpful for his metabolic health. One night, around four years after his diagnosis of T2D, he collapsed on his way to the bathroom. He had suffered a major stroke and sadly did not recover. Artery disease is a major accompaniment of T2D, but at the age of eighty-two some would view his passing as age-related and not unexpected. There is no way of knowing whether T2D shortened his life, or if metformin and blood pressure medication may have extended it.

Benjamin

Benjamin, fifty-six, has reasonably stable T2D, though dietary discipline has proved difficult and he struggles with his mood. Worries about having T2D have affected his quality of life and put a strain on his marriage. With four years left before mandatory retirement (age sixty for air traffic controllers), Benjamin worries he might need insulin in future which would prevent him working. He worries about unravelling psychologically without work. Though his T2D is reasonably stable, he feels his future is uncertain. He has engaged with psychological help which was initiated from a work medical review. Benjamin tends to suppress his emotions but has been able to work on his distressing thoughts and learn to be more compassionate towards himself. Occupational health also raised the option of working in a different role after sixty, which gives him hope.

Nandita

Nandita stopped working as a music teacher at fifty-five, around the time she started insulin. She had neuropathy which affected the way her hands felt and functioned. She ruminated about T2D, having damaged nerves, snack guilt (mainly biscuits) and missing medical appointments. She became quite apathetic. Her healthcare team arranged for her to see a psychological therapist who encouraged her to develop her interest in music composition software. She went back to work part-time helping students in the school music studio. She also joined a T2D support group, which gave her a new social outlet. By following her therapist's advice and using self-help around behavioural activation, her mood improved. She found the group emotionally supportive and picked up some helpful tips on snacking! Through being more active, life is starting to feel different.

Colin

In his early sixties, Colin faced T2D, a heart attack and depression, alongside a threat of redundancy. CBT helped address his depression and uncovered erectile dysfunction. Successful management of this problem was a major component in Colin's recovery. Erectile dysfunction is such an accepted part of T2D, indeed just getting older, that many men will play down its role in their life. This can have major negative impacts for the individual and be damaging to relationships if not managed openly. A year or so after his diagnoses, Colin was self-managing his T2D and his mood (using the CBT strategies he had learned), enjoying his life and engaging in the challenge of attempting reversal of his T2D. It would be difficult to overstate the impact that CBT had in helping him turn his life around.

Alan

A policeman in his early forties, Alan's weight and blood pressure had risen, and he was diagnosed with NAFLD. Next stop T2D, you would think. He had thought that being an all-round exerciser and jogging twenty or more miles a week would always keep him healthy. He would joke, 'I run so that I can eat chips.' A few years later, Alan left the police force, working part-time in a much less stressful job. He had eventually accepted the advice of friends and colleagues, but especially his wife, to reflect on the potential risks of working hard and playing hard. He adjusted his diet, reduced his alcohol and found his weight dropping despite running less. Limiting his carbohydrates – including his chips – helped him to reverse his NAFLD and (probably) prevent T2D.

Summary of key points from the book

We'll close with a short summary of the book's main messages. These notes can serve as a summary of your book experience or a 'go-to' for any key reminders. We think they are the things that matter!

The main types of diabetes, T1D and T2D, are very different. Any disturbance in the function of insulin will impact blood glucose. If insulin disappears quickly, as in T1D, the rise in blood glucose and accompanying illness is rapid. When insulin becomes slowly and progressively impaired, as in T2D, the rise in blood glucose is relatively slow and the symptoms of hyperglycaemia can feel mild. Unfortunately, the accompanying changes in the body are not mild. Rising weight, liver fat, blood pressure and glucose, and artery disease are affecting now, in one way or another, the majority of adults around the world. Underpinning these (and other) conditions is dysregulated or impaired insulin – whether it be insulin excess, resistance, or absence. Insulin has become broken and we have to fix it.

T2D develops slowly but it can be addressed **FAST**!

Food. We can be fairly sure that many of us are putting the wrong fuel/food in our 'engine'. The issue may be partly one of balance – eating too many carbohydrates (especially sugar/fructose) – or it may be too much energy (food) overall, and the two things may be linked. The brain and liver are so connected in metabolism, and brain chemistry both drives and responds to changes in the food that we seek and eat. We have become easy grazers on sugar-rich snacks and ultra-processed foods and drinks.

When we eat the right food for us, problems with metabolism are prevented or reversed; if we go back to eating the wrong food, those problems reappear. Insulin-linked or metabolic diseases can all follow from this simple misfuelling of the body. It looks increasingly like modern food and eating habits are driving the world's leading health problems.

The right dietary approach for you is one that helps, reverses and/or maintains remission of your T2D. It will help you to lose and stabilise both your weight and liver fat. No single dietary approach is likely to work well for every single person. Very low-calorie diets can reverse T2D well but may be harder to sustain long-term. Low-carbohydrate diets can reverse and probably maintain remission better. Moving from low-calorie eating for reversal to low-carbohydrate eating makes perfect sense in the longer term. A nutrient-dense wholefood or Mediterranean diet might also work (short- and long-term) for more people than not.

Intermittent fasting might be a more sustainable way of restricting calories. Eating mindfully, shopping more thought-fully, cooking to freeze and cupboard/snack management can all help with managing food issues.

The fat fear conundrum has to be addressed by anyone engaged in low-carbohydrate eating. We can only repeat that, while science cannot exclude risk from eating saturated fat, a rethink is taking place and many now think that risk has been overstated, or indeed may be near absent. The risks meantime from T2D are large and very real. If managing T2D involves eating more fat, the risk equation favours doing it, with eating more fat from non-animal sources a way of 'covering options'!

Activity and sleep. These are the twin supports of healthy metabolism, and being active like our ancestors undoubtedly contributed to their lack of modern disease. However, when an active lifestyle is out of reach, timed *regular* exercise is much better than none. A moderate to high level of exercise can improve insulin function, prevent T2D and improve its management. If weight loss is needed, it's best to achieve that through diet first. Losing fat means the body is able to release energy, making exercise easier and more effective. The rightful place of exercise is 'on the shoulder' of healthy eating.

The health benefits of sleep are less well-known than those of diet and exercise, but science has revealed a rich vein of activity – of repair, maintenance and 'system resetting' (including memory) when we sleep. Good sleep duration varies between individuals but six to eight hours is near the mark. It's also better to allow the body's internal clocks to follow those of the natural day/night cycles of our environment. Rotational shift work is especially challenging to the body's metabolic processes, which are themselves 'clock-driven'. Medication (including alcohol) does not bring with it the benefits of normal sleep, and is best avoided if sleep is a big problem. In health, improving sleep sits 'on the other shoulder' of eating well.

Tension/stress. Occasional and intermittent stress produces short-lived physical responses within the body which help us to deal with that stress. When stress is severe and persistent, however, nervous and hormonal responses which are adaptive and healthy in the short term become harmful and damaging in the longer term. The stress hormone system, linking the brain and adrenal glands, is overworked, and one consequence of this is an impairment of glucose and insulin metabolism.

The more severe the stress, the greater its impact on the control of glucose – and mental illness such as depression raises the risk of T2D twofold; severe mental illnesses such as schizophrenia raise that risk much more. Mental illness also means that a person is much less likely to look after themselves – to eat healthily and keep active, for example. These things mean that mental health problems can bring a sense of swimming against the tide with T2D, and need to be addressed as a priority.

FAST embodies the causes of T2D, and is also a call to action. Whilst getting food right is the priority for us all, better sleep, being active and managing stress/mental health problems all play their part. **FAST is our reminder that we are all 'joined up'.**

Self-managing and reducing risks

Artery disease is the commonest cause of death worldwide and one of its biggest risk factors is T2D. Reversing T2D helps to near-normalise the risk from that. Improving control of blood glucose without reversal helps to lower risk of artery disease, though by a much lesser degree. Smoking is equally damaging to arteries and should also be addressed to keep those risks low.

Self-managing means looking more widely at risk factors for artery disease, avoiding drugs which might increase risk, and managing stress and alcohol. We can help ourselves by identifying links between potential risks we can measure – the main one being blood pressure – and what we do, such as how much we eat and drink and when. Sleep, exercise, weight, mood and stress can all be self-monitored (in a diary) to examine for connections between them, and with measures like blood pressure, glucose (or HbA1c) and with wellbeing. Monitoring with support almost certainly improves what's being monitored and overall health.

T2D is in transition

Cell science is teaching us how and why our cells respond to hormones like insulin, which in turn links those responses to how we live, especially the food we eat. We know that meta-bolic diseases like T2D are probably linked to many cancers and that both develop more readily when the body exists in a state of low-level inflammation, which itself can be impacted by food choices. It's looking more and more like the signa-ture diseases of our age may share a dietary basis. Once we understand better how to measure markers of susceptibility to disease – currently a little crude at the frontline of healthcare – new dietary therapies targeted to individuals, to both prevent and treat disease, may appear. The concept of 'one diet fits all' will then seem even more out-of-date.

We saw that the chemistry of pregnancy and epigenetics may be throwing light on why T2D (and related conditions) are surging beyond expectations. Women with T2D, GDM and those who are significantly overweight transmit a much higher risk of T2D and artery disease to their offspring throughout *those children's* lives, and possibly the generation beyond. Teenage girls and young women at risk of future T2D in particular need to be aware of the risks of such heightened transmission. Women already with T2D should ideally plan pregnancy and keep glucose as low as possible *before* getting pregnant. Up until very recently this was not happening, at least in the UK, though there are now encouraging signs of change for the better.

Although pregnancy transmission suggests a mechanism for disease escalation, it also helps our understanding of T2D, and as with the work on reversal, it offers hope for the future. T2D and GDM are preventable and the risks from diabetes in pregnancy and epigenetic impacts can be modified by improved management of blood glucose.

These days it can look as though we are making a mess of our environments – both the external one involving our planet and the internal one involving our own bodies. The two things may not be completely separate, but as individuals we can only directly control our internal environment.

Last pause to reflect

If you are one of the half a billion people with T2D or the billion or more who are at risk of T2D, what choices can *you* make to stay healthy?

You would most probably choose a diet and lifestyle that would make you or keep you well rather than unwell. But being able to decide means knowing what to do and having the means to do it. A simple choice is never quite as easy as it sounds – we know that healthy food can be difficult to access or afford in some parts of the world. And yet in many countries we can see it's healthier to live a more basic, rural 'gatherer' if not 'hunter' lifestyle. Living cheaply in that sense is healthy. Living in cities, which is increasingly the norm, it can feel a lot harder to stay healthy on a low income.

However hard it is to eat well, it is always *possible* to a degree, and where there is scope there is hope! Belief is maybe the key to changing your own personal way of life, and beliefs are part of being human. Our knowledge and experience feed them and can amend them. Oftentimes our beliefs help us, but sometimes they trap us. When things are not working, we question whether we are 'doing it right' or 'trying hard enough'. Maybe 'Are we doing the right thing?' is sometimes a better question to ask.

Beliefs and motivation to act are strongly bound together. Finding the deep motivation to help change for the better is a big part of getting to grips with T2D. Think of the motivation of the people in the book, how that differed and how it might have affected their journeys (so far).

Though the last two decades can feel gloomy from a numbers perspective, new knowledge suggests that this can now be an optimistic period for T2D. As individuals we can reach out for the knowledge we need to help us change, but we also need to look inwards to find the motivation to fuel – and refuel – that change. Both are needed to help us find what works.

Many people out there have found what works for them – could you join them?

Appendix 1: References and Further Reading

Introduction

Khan, M.A.B., Hashim, M.J. et al. (2020). Epidemiology of type 2 diabetes: global burden of disease and forecasted trends. *Journal of Epidemiology and Global Health*, 10(1): 107–11.

Sun, H., Saeedi, P. et al. (2022). IDF Diabetes Atlas: global, regional and country-level diabetes prevalence estimates for 2021 and projections for 2045. *Diabetes Research and Clinical Practice*, 183: 109119.

Wang, L., Peng, W. et al. (2021). Prevalence and treatment of diabetes in China, 2013–2018. *JAMA*, 326(24): 2498–506.

Chapter 1

Diabetes UK (2019). Fact sheet 25-02-2019. Retrieved from: www.diabetes.org.uk/about_us/news/new-stats-people-living-with-diabetes.

Khademvatan, K., Alinejad, V. et al. (2014). Survey of the relationship between metabolic syndrome and myocardial infarction in hospitals of Urmia University of Medical Sciences. *Global Journal of Health Science*, 6(7): 58–65.

Kyle, R.G., Wills, J. et al. (2017). Obesity prevalence among healthcare professionals in England: a cross-sectional study using the Health Survey for England. *BMJ Open*, 7e018498.

Saklayen, M.G. (2018). The global epidemic of the metabolic syndrome. *Current Hypertension Reports*, 20(2): 12.

UK Government Office for Health Improvement and Disparities (2022). Obesity profile (updated July 2022). Retrieved from: www.gov.uk/government/statistics/obesity-profile-update-july-2022.

UK Government Office for Health Improvement and Disparities (2022). Childhood obesity: patterns and trends (updated 5 April 2022). Retrieved from: https://fingertips.phe.org.uk/profile/national-child-measurement-programme.

UK National Institute for Clinical Excellence (NICE). Clinical knowledge summaries: non-alcoholic fatty liver disease – prevalence (October 2021). Retrieved from: https://cks.nice.org.uk/topics/non-alcoholic-fatty-liver-disease-nafld/background-information/prevalence/.

UK NHS Digital (2021–22). NHS national diabetes audit. Retrieved from: https://digital.nhs.uk/data-and-information/publications/statistical/national-diabetes-audit/nda-core-e4-21-22/nda-core-e4-21-22.

UK NHS Digital (2021–22). Quality and outcomes framework. Practice-based data on diabetes prevalence. Retrieved from: https://digital.nhs.uk/data-and-information/publications/statistical/quality-and-outcomes-framework-achievement-prevalence-and-exceptions-data/2021-22.

Uppin, A.M., Badiger, R.H. et al. (2020). Assessment of incidence rate and prognosis of metabolic syndrome among acute myocardial infarction: a longitudinal study. *International Journal of Advances in Medicine*, 7(2): 267–71.

World Health Organization (2021). Fact sheet on obesity and overweight (June 2021). Retrieved from: www.who.int/news-room/fact-sheets/detail/obesity-and-overweight.

Chapter 2

Alberti, K.G.M.M., Eckel, R.H. et al. (2009). Harmonizing the metabolic syndrome. A joint interim statement of the International Diabetes Federation Task Force on Epidemiology and Prevention; National Heart, Lung, and Blood Institute; American Heart Association; World Heart Federation; International Atherosclerosis Society; and International Association for the Study of Obesity. *Circulation*, 120(16): 1640–5.

Freese, J., Klement, R.J. et al. (2017). The sedentary (r)evolution: have we lost our metabolic flexibility? *F1000Research*, 2 October, 6: 1787.

Gallicia-Garcia, U., Benito-Vicente, A. et al. (2020). Pathophysiology of type 2 diabetes mellitus. *International Journal of Molecular Sciences*, 21(17): 6275.

Gordon, L. & Levkowitz, G. (2021). Through the open window: how does the brain talk to the body? *Frontiers for Young Minds*, 9: 534184 (Source of Figure 2.1.)

Kolb, H., Kempf, K. et al. (2020). Insulin: too much of a good thing is bad. *BMC Medicine*, 18(1): 224.

Mitra, S., De, A. & Chowdhury, A. (2020). Epidemiology of non-alcoholic and alcoholic fatty liver diseases. *Translational Gastroenterology and Hepatology*, 5: 16.

Pories, W.J. & Dohm, G.L. (2012). Diabetes: have we got it all wrong? Hyperinsulinism as the culprit: surgery provides the evidence. *Diabetes Care*, 35(12): 2438–42.

Smith, G.I., Mittendorfer, B. & Klein, S. (2019). Metabolically healthy obesity: facts and fantasies. *Journal of Clinical Investigation*, 129(10): 3978–89.

Tabák, A.G., Jokela, M. et al. (2009). Trajectories of glycaemia, insulin sensitivity, and insulin secretion before diagnosis of type 2 diabetes: an analysis from the Whitehall II study. *The Lancet*, 373(9682): 2215–21.

Taylor, R. & Barnes, A.C. (2018). Translating aetiological insight into sustainable management of type 2 diabetes. *Diabetologia*, 61(2): 273–83.

Taylor, R. (2012). *Banting memorial lecture*. Reversing the twin cycles of type 2 diabetes. *Diabetic Medicine*, 30(3): 267–75.

UK National Institute for Health and Care Excellence (NICE) (2021). Non-alcoholic fatty liver disease (NAFLD): prevalence. *Clinical Knowledge Summaries* (rev. October 2021). Retrieved from: https://cks.nice.org.uk/topics/non-alcoholic-fatty-liver-disease-nafld/background-information/prevalence/.

Chapter 3

Belvediri Murri, M., Ekkekakis, P. et al. (2018). Physical exercise in major depression: reducing the mortality gap while improving clinical outcomes. *Frontiers in Psychiatry*, 9, article 762.

Careau, V., Halsey, L.G. et al. (2021). Energy compensation and adiposity in humans. *Current Biology*, 31(20): 4659–66.e2.

Catenacci, V.A. & Wyatt, H.R. (2007). The role of physical activity in producing and maintaining weight loss. *Nature Clinical Practice Endocrinology & Metabolism*, 3(7): 518–29.

Department of Health and Social Care (2019). UK Chief Medical Officers' physical activity guidelines, 7 September. Retrieved from: https://assets.publishing.service.gov.uk/government/uploads/system/uploads/attachment_data/file/832868/uk-chief-medical-officers-physical-activity-guidelines.pdf.

Ensari, I., Greenlee, T.A. et al. (2015). Meta-analysis of acute exercise effects on state anxiety: an update of randomized controlled trials over the past 25 years. *Depression and Anxiety*, 32(8): 624–34.

Gaesser, G.A. & Angardi, S.S. (2021). Obesity treatment: weight loss versus increasing fitness and physical activity for reducing health risks. *iScience*, 24(10): 102995.

Gilmore, C.P. (1977). Taking exercise to heart. *New York Times*, 27 March, p. 211.

Liu, J.-X., Zhu, L. et al. (2019). Effectiveness of high-intensity interval training on glycemic control and cardiorespiratory fitness in patients with type 2 diabetes: a systematic review and meta-analysis. *Aging Clinical and Experimental Research*, 31(5): 575–93.

Memme, J.M., Erlich, A.T. et al. (2021). Exercise and mitochondrial health. *Journal of Physiology*, 599(3): 803–17.

Metcalf, B.S., Hosking, J. et al. (2010). Fatness leads to inactivity, but inactivity does not lead to fatness: a longitudinal study in children (EarlyBird 45). *Archives of Disease in Childhood*, 96: 942–7.

Pontzer, H., Wood, B.M. & Raichlen, D.A. (2018). Hunter-gatherers as models in public health. *Obesity Reviews*, 19(Suppl. 1): 24–35.

Reid, H., Ridout, A.J. et al. (2022). Benefits outweigh the risks: a consensus statement on the risks of physical activity for people living with long-term conditions. *British Journal of Sports Medicine*, 56: 427–38.

Singh, B., Olds, T. et al. (2022). Effectiveness of physical activity interventions for improving depression, anxiety and distress: an overview of systematic reviews. *British Journal of Sports Medicine*, 16 February 2023: 1–10.

Smith, A.D., Crippa, A. et al. (2016). Physical activity and incident type 2 diabetes mellitus: a systematic review and dose-response meta-analysis of prospective cohort studies. *Diabetologia*, 59(12): 2527–45.

Tipton, C.M. (2014). The history of 'Exercise is Medicine' in ancient civilizations. *Advances in Physiology Education*, 38(2): 109–17.

Chapter 4

Ahmadian, N., Hejazi, S. et al. (2018). Tau pathology of Alzheimer's disease: possible role of sleep deprivation. *Basic and Clinical Neuro-science*, 9(5): 307–16.

Anderson, K. (2023). *How to Beat Insomnia and Sleep Problems*. London: Robinson.

Anothaisintawee, T., Reutrakul, S. et al. (2016). Sleep disturbances compared to traditional risk factors for diabetes development: systematic review and meta-analysis. *Sleep Medicine Reviews*, 30: 11–24.

Antza, C., Kostopoulos, G. et al. (2021). The links between sleep duration, obesity and type 2 diabetes mellitus. *Journal of Endocrinology*, 252(2): 125–41.

Benjafield, A.V., Ayas, N.T. et al. (2019). Estimation of the global prevalence and burden of obstructive sleep apnoea: a literature-based analysis. *Lancet Respiratory Medicine*, 7(8): 687–98.

Chu, Y., Oh, Y. et al. (2023). Dose-response analysis of smart-phone usage and self-reported sleep quality: a systematic review and meta-analysis of observational studies. *Journal of Clinical Sleep Medicine*, 19(3): 621–30.

Gottlieb, D.J. & Punjabi, N.M. (2020). Diagnosis and management of obstructive sleep apnea: a review. *JAMA,* 323(14): 1389–400.

Leong, R.L.F., Lau, T. et al. (2023). Influence of mid-afternoon nap duration and sleep parameters on memory encoding, mood, processing speed, and vigilance. *Sleep*, 46(4): zsad025.

Mallon, L., Broman, J.E. & Hetta, J. (2005). High incidence of diabetes in men with sleep complaints or short sleep duration: a 12-year follow-up study of a middle-aged population. *Diabetes Care*, 28(11): 2762–7.

Mantua, J. & Spencer, R.M.C. (2017). Exploring the nap paradox: are mid-day sleep bouts a friend or foe? *Sleep Medicine*, 37: 88–97.

Quinn, D. (2011). *The Holy*. Hanover, NH: Steerforth Press.

Reutrakul, S. & Van Cauter, E. (2014). Interactions between sleep, circadian function, and glucose metabolism: implications for risk and severity of diabetes. *Annals of the New York Academy of Sciences*, 1311: 151–73.

Schipper, S.B.J., Van Veen, M.M. et al. (2021). Sleep disorders in people with type 2 diabetes and associated health outcomes: a review of the literature. *Diabetologia*, 64: 2367–77.

Shan, Z., Li, Y. et al. (2018). Rotating night shift work and adherence to unhealthy lifestyle in predicting risk of type 2 diabetes: results from two large US cohorts of female nurses. *BMJ*, 363: k4641.

Shan, Z., Ma, H. et al. (2015). Sleep duration and risk of type 2 diabetes: a meta-analysis of prospective studies. *Diabetes Care*, 38(3): 529–37.

Shapiro, C. (2011). The patterns of sleep disorders and circadian rhythm disruptions in children and adolescents with fetal alcohol spectrum disorders. Adapted from Lin, V.W., Cardenas, D.D. et al. (2003). *Spinal Cord Medicine: Principles and Practice*. New York: Demos Medical Publishing.

Sharma, S. & Kavuru, M. (2010). Sleep and metabolism: an overview. *International Journal of Endocrinology*, 2010: 270832.

Stevens, A. (1997). *Private Myths: Dreams and Dreaming*. Cambridge MA: Harvard University Press.

Tefft, B.C. (2018). Acute sleep deprivation and culpable motor vehicle crash involvement. *Sleep*, 41(10): 30239905.

Vetter, C., Dashti, H.S. et al. (2018). Night shift work, genetic risk, and type 2 diabetes in the UK Biobank. *Diabetes Care*, 41(4): 762–9.

Walker, M.P. & Stickgold, R. (2006). Sleep, memory, and plasticity. *Annual Review of Psychology*, 57: 139–66.

Chapter 5

Athinarayanan, S.J., Adams, R.N. et al. (2019). Long-term effects of a novel continuous remote care intervention including nutritional ketosis for the management of type 2 diabetes: a 2-year non-randomized clinical trial. *Frontiers in Endocrinology*, 10: 348.

Berg, A. (2020). Untold stories of living with a bariatric body: long-term experiences of weight-loss surgery. *Sociology of Health & Illness*, 42: 217–31.

Coulman, K.D., MacKichan, F. et al. (2020). Patients' experiences of life after bariatric surgery and follow-up care: a qualitative study. *BMJ Open*, 10: e035013.

Diabetes UK (2021). Position statement: remission in adults with type 2 diabetes. Retrieved from: https://diabetes-resources-production.s3.eu-west-1.amazonaws.com/resources-s3/public/2021-08/DIABETES %20UK%20UPDATED%20POSITION%20STATEMENT%20 ON%20REMISSION%20IN%20ADULTS%20-%20FINAL_0.pdf.

Esposito, K., Maiorino, M.A. et al. (2014). The effects of a Mediterranean diet on the need for diabetes drugs and remission of newly diagnosed type 2 diabetes: follow-up of a randomized trial. *Diabetes Care*, 37(7): 1824–30.

Gregg, E.W., Chen, H. et al. & Look AHEAD Research Group (2012). Association of an intensive lifestyle intervention with remission of type 2 diabetes. JAMA, 308(23): 2489–96.

Hallberg, S. (2018). Reversing type 2 diabetes starts with ignoring the guidelines: education from Dr Sarah Hallberg's TEDx talk. *British Journal of Sports Medicine*, 52: 869–71. Retrieved from: www.youtube.com/watch?v=da1vvigy5tQ.

International Federation for the Surgery of Obesity and Metabolic Disorders (IFSO) (2022). *7th IFSO Global Registry Report 2022*. Retrieved from: www.ifso.com/pdf/ifso-7th-registry-report-2022.pdf.

Lean, M., Leslie, W.S. et al. (2019). Durability of a primary care-led weight-management intervention for remission of type 2 diabetes: 2-year results of the DiRECT open-label, cluster-randomised trial. *Lancet Diabetes & Endocrinology*, 7(5): 344–55.

Lim, R., Beekley, A. et al. (2018). Early and late complications of bariatric operation. *Trauma Surgery & Acute Care Open*, 3: e000219.

Lupoli, R., Lembo, E. et al. (2017). Bariatric surgery and long-term nutritional issues. *World Journal of Diabetes*, 8(11): 464–74.

O'Dea, K. (2016). The Aboriginal hunter-gatherer lifestyle: lessons for chronic disease prevention. *Pathology*, 48(Suppl. 1): S14.

Sinclair, P., Docherty, N. & le Roux, C.W. (2018). Metabolic effects of bariatric surgery. *Clinical Chemistry*, 64(1): 72–81.

Taheri, S., Zaghloul, H. et al. (2020). Effect of intensive lifestyle intervention on bodyweight and glycaemia in early type 2 diabetes (DIADEM-I): an open-label, parallel-group, randomised controlled trial. *Lancet Diabetes & Endocrinology*, 8(6): 477–89.

Taylor, R., Ramachandran, A. et al. (2021). Nutritional basis of type 2 diabetes remission. *BMJ*, 374: n1449.

Tsilingiris, D., Koliaki, C. & Kokkinos, A. (2019). Remission of type 2 diabetes mellitus after bariatric surgery: fact or fiction? *International Journal of Environmental Research and Public Health,* 16(17): 3171.

UK All Party Parliamentary Group (APPG) for Diabetes (2018). *Reversing Type 2 Diabetes*, 8 August. Retrieved from: https://diabetes appg.files.wordpress.com/2019/08/2018-reversing-type-2-diabetes-snap-report.pdf.

UK National Bariatric Surgery Registry (NBSR) (2020). *NBSR 3rd Registry Report 2020*. Retrieved from: https://e-dendrite.com/ Publishing/Reports/Bariatric/NBSR2020.pdf.

White, M.G., Shaw, J.A.M. & Taylor, R. (2016). Type 2 diabetes: the pathologic basis of reversible beta-cell dysfunction. *Diabetes Care*, 39: 2080–8.

Chapter 6

Ahima, R.S. & Antwi, D.A. (2008). Brain regulation of appetite and satiety. *Endocrinology and Metabolism Clinics of North America*, 37(4): 811–23.

Ahmad, S., Demler, O.V. et al. (2020). Association of the Mediterranean diet with onset of diabetes in the women's health study. *JAMA Network Open*, 3(11): e2025466. Retrieved from: https://jama-network.com/journals/jamanetworkopen/fullarticle/2773099.

Albosta, M. & Bakke, J. (2021). Intermittent fasting: is there a role in the treatment of diabetes? A review of the literature and guide for primary care physicians. *Clinical Diabetes and Endocrinology*, 7: 3.

Astrup, A., Magkos, F. et al. (2020). Saturated fats and health: a reassessment and proposal for food-based recommendations. *Journal of the American College of Cardiology*, 76(7): 844–57.

Baker, P., Machado, P. et al. (2020). Ultra-processed foods and the nutrition transition: global, regional and national trends, food systems transformations and political economy drivers. *Obesity Reviews*, 21(12): e13126.

Brown, A., McArdle, P. et al. (2022). Dietary strategies for remission of type 2 diabetes: a narrative review. *Journal of Human Nutrition and Dietetics*, 35(1): 165–78.

Buljeta, I., Pichler, A. et al. (2023). Beneficial effects of red wine polyphenols on human health: comprehensive review. *Current Issues in Molecular Biology*, 45: 782–98.

De Souza, R.J., Mente, A. et al. (2015). Intake of saturated and trans unsaturated fatty acids and risk of all cause mortality, cardiovascular disease, and type 2 diabetes: systematic review and meta-analysis of observational studies. *BMJ*, 351: h3978.

Dunn, C., Haubenreiser, M. et al. (2018). Mindfulness approaches and weight loss, weight maintenance, and weight regain. *Current Obesity Reports*, 7: 37–49.

Estruch, R., Ross, E. et al. for the PREDIMED Study Investigators (2018). Primary prevention of cardiovascular disease with a

Mediterranean diet supplemented with extra-virgin olive oil or nuts. *New England Journal of Medicine*, 378: e34.

Forouhi, N., Misra, A. et al. (2018). Dietary and nutritional approaches for prevention and management of type 2 diabetes. *BMJ*, 361: k2234.

Forouhi, N.G., Krauss, R.M. et al. (2018). Dietary fat and cardiometabolic health: evidence, controversies, and consensus for guidance. *BMJ*, 361: k2139.

GBD 2016 Alcohol Collaborators (2018). Alcohol use and burden for 195 countries and territories, 1990–2016: a systematic analysis for the Global Burden of Disease Study 2016. *The Lancet*, 392: 1015–35.

Grajower, M.M. & Horne, B.D. (2019). Clinical management of intermittent fasting in patients with diabetes mellitus. *Nutrients*, 11(4): 873.

Grandjean, P. (2016). Paracelsus revisited: the dose concept in a complex world. *Basic & Clinical Pharmacology & Toxicology*, 119(2): 126–32. Epub 24 June 2016.

Hurst, Y. & Fukuda, H. (2018). Effects of changes in eating speed on obesity in patients with diabetes: a secondary analysis of longitudinal health check-up data. *BMJ Open*, 8: e019589.

Kamilla, L., Silva, C.P. et al. (2022). Time-restricted eating and exercise training improve HbA1c and body composition in women with overweight/obesity: a randomized controlled trial. *Cell Metabolism*, 34(10): 1457–71.e4.

Liu, A.G., Ford, N.A. et al. (2017). A healthy approach to dietary fats: understanding the science and taking action to reduce consumer confusion. *Nutritional Journal*, 16, article 53.

Ludwig, D.S., Apovian, C.M. et al. (2022). Competing paradigms of obesity pathogenesis: energy balance versus carbohydrate-insulin models. *European Journal of Clinical Nutrition*, 76: 1209–21.

Luiten, C., Steenhuis, I. et al. (2015). Ultra-processed foods have the worst nutrient profile, yet they are the most available packaged products in a sample of New Zealand supermarkets. *Public Health Nutrition*, 19(3): 530–8.

Lustig, R. (2008). Which comes first? The obesity or the insulin? The behavior or the biochemistry? *Journal of Pediatrics*, 152(5): 601–2.

Lustig, R.H. (2020). Ultra-processed food: addictive, toxic, and ready for regulation. *Nutrients*, 12(11): 3401.

MacLean, P.S., Blundell, J.E. et al. (2017). Biological control of appetite: a daunting complexity. *Obesity*, 25(Suppl. 1): S8–S16.

Mardinoglu, A., Wu, H. et al. (2018). An integrated understanding of the rapid metabolic benefits of a carbohydrate-restricted diet on hepatic steatosis in humans. *Cell Metabolism*, 27(3): 559–71.

Martín-Peláez, S., Fito, M. & Castaner, O. (2020). Mediterranean diet effects on type 2 diabetes prevention, disease progression, and related mechanisms. A review. *Nutrients*, 12(8): 2236.

Milenkovic, T., Bozhinovska, N. et al. (2021). Mediterranean diet and type 2 diabetes mellitus: a perpetual inspiration for the scientific world. A review. *Nutrients*, 13(4): 1307.

Miller, C.K. (2017). Mindful eating with diabetes. *DiabetesSpectrum*, 30(2): pp. 89–94.

Rauber, F., da Costa Louzada, M.L. et al. (2018). Ultra-processed foods and excessive free sugar intake in the UK: a nationally representative cross-sectional study. *BMJ Open*, 9: e027546.

Sarsangi, P., Salehi-Abargouei, A. et al. (2022). Association between adherence to the Mediterranean diet and risk of type 2 diabetes: an updated systematic review and dose–response meta-analysis of prospective cohort studies. *Advances in Nutrition*, 13(5): 1787–98.

Softic, S., Stanhope, K.L. et al. (2020). Fructose and hepatic insulin resistance. *Critical Reviews in Clinical Laboratory Sciences*, 57(5): 308–22.

Taskinen, M.R., Packard, J. & Boren, J. (2019). Dietary fructose and the metabolic syndrome. *Nutrients*, 11(9): 1987.

Taubes, G. (2013). The science of obesity: what do we really know about what makes us fat? *BMJ*, 346: f1050.

Temple, N.J. (2018). Fat, sugar, whole grains and heart disease: 50 years of confusion. *Nutrients*, 10(1): 39.

UK NHS (n.d.). The Eatwell Guide. Retrieved from: www.nhs.uk/live-well/eat-well/food-guidelines-and-food-labels/the-eatwell-guide (page last reviewed 29 November 2022).

UK Scientific Advisory Committee on Nutrition (SACN) (2021). Lower carbohydrate diets for adults with type 2 diabetes. © Crown copyright 2021. Retrieved from: www.gov.uk/government/groups/scientific-advisory-committee-on-nutrition.

Unwin, D. & Unwin, J. (2014). Low-carbohydrate diet to achieve weight loss and improve HbA1c in type 2 diabetes and pre-diabetes: experience from one general practice. *Practical Diabetes*, 31(2): 76–9.

US Department of Agriculture & US Department of Health and Human Services (2020). *Dietary Guidelines for Americans, 2020–2025* (9th edn). Retrieved from: www.dietaryguidelines.gov/sites/default/files/2020-12/Dietary_Guidelines_for_Americans_2020-2025.pdf.

Valk, R., Hammill, J. & Grip, J. (2022). Saturated fat: villain and bogeyman in the development of cardiovascular disease? *European Journal of Preventive Cardiology*, 29(18): 2312–21.

Weeratunga, P., Jayasinghe, S. et al. (2014). Per capita sugar consumption and prevalence of diabetes mellitus – global and regional associations. *BMC Public Health*, 14: 186.

Westman, E.C. (2002). Is dietary carbohydrate essential for human nutrition? *American Journal of Clinical Nutrition*, 75(5): 951–3.

Wheatley, S.D., Deakin, T.A. et al. (2021). Low carbohydrate dietary approaches for people with type 2 diabetes – a narrative review. *Frontiers in Nutrition*, 15 July; Sec. Clinical Nutrition, 8.

Yamaji, T., Mikami, T. et al. (2018). Gobbling your food is the risk factor of obesity and metabolic syndrome. *European Heart Journal*, 39(Suppl. 1).

Chapter 7

Ariel, H. & Cooke, J.P. (2019). Cardiovascular risk of proton pump inhibitors. *Methodist DeBakey Cardiovascular Journal*, 15(3): 214–19.

Bally, M., Dendukuri, N. et al. (2017). Risk of acute myocardial infarction with NSAIDs in real world use: Bayesian meta-analysis of individual patient data. *BMJ*, 357: j1909.

Bøtker, H.E. & Møller, N. (2013). ON NO – the continuing story of nitric oxide, diabetes, and cardiovascular disease. *Diabetes*, 62(8): 2645–7.

British Heart Foundation (2022). Can meditation help people with heart disease? *Heart Matters*. Retrieved from: www.bhf.org.uk/inform ationsupport/heart-matters-magazine/wellbeing/meditation-and-mindfulness.

Campagna, D., Alamo, A. et al. (2019). Smoking and diabetes: dangerous liaisons and confusing relationships. *Diabetology and Metabolic Syndrome*, 11: 85.

Crandall, J.P., Mather, K. et al. (2017). Statin use and risk of developing diabetes: results from the Diabetes Prevention Program. *BMJ Open Diabetes Research & Care*, 5: e000438.

Einarson, T.R., Acs, A. et al. (2018). Prevalence of cardiovascular disease in type 2 diabetes: a systematic literature review of scientific evidence from across the world in 2007–2017. *Cardiovascular Diabetology*, 17: 83.

Elnaem, M.H., Mohamed, M.H.N. et al. (2017). Statin therapy prescribing for patients with type 2 diabetes mellitus: a review of current evidence and challenges. *Journal of Pharmacy and Bioallied Sciences*, 9(2): 80–7.

Esposito, K., Maiorino, M.G. et al. (2010). Determinants of female sexual dysfunction in type 2 diabetes. *International Journal* of Impotence Research, 22: 179–84.

Joseph, J.J. & Golden, S.H. (2017). Cortisol dysregulation: the bidirectional link between stress, depression, and type 2 diabetes mellitus. *Annals of the New York Academy of Sciences*, 1391(1): 20–34. Epub 17 October 2016.

Laakso, M. & Kuusisto, J. (2014). Insulin resistance and hyperglycaemia in cardiovascular disease development. *Nature Reviews Endocrinology*, 10: 293–302.

Nielsen, R.E., Banner, J. & Jensen, S.E. (2021). Cardiovascular disease in patients with severe mental illness. *Nature Reviews Cardiology*, 18: 136–45.

Ohishi, M. (2018). Hypertension with diabetes mellitus: physiology and pathology. *Hypertension Research*, 41(6): 389–93. Epub 19 March 2018.

Ormazabal, V., Nair, S. et al. (2018). Association between insulin resistance and the development of cardiovascular disease. *Cardiovascular Diabetology*, 17: 122.

Roth, G., Mensah, G. et al. (2020). Global burden of cardiovascular diseases and risk factors, 1990–2019. *Journal of the American College of Cardiology*, 76(25): 2982–3021.

Shindel, A.W. and Lue, T.F. (2000). Sexual dysfunction in diabetes. In: Feingold, K.R., Anawalt, B., Blackman, M.R. et al. (eds), *Endotext* [internet]. South Dartmouth, MA: MDText.com, Inc. (updated June 2021). Retrieved from: www.ncbi.nlm.nih.gov/books/NBK279101/.

Stehouwer, C.D.A. (2018). Microvascular dysfunction and hyperglycemia: a vicious cycle with widespread consequences. *Diabetes*, 67(9): 1729–41.

Steptoe, A. & Kivimäki, M. (2012). Stress and cardiovascular disease. *Nature Reviews Cardiology*, 9: 360–70.

United Kingdom Prospective Diabetes Study (UKPDS) 1977–1997, summary of the trial, component studies and legacy effects – 2022. Includes an interview with one of the principal investigators Professor Rury Holman. Diabetes Trials Unit, Oxford Centre for Diabetes, Endocrinology and Metabolism. Retrieved from: www.dtu.ox.ac.uk/ukpds.

Weller, R.B. (2016). Sunlight has cardiovascular benefits independently of vitamin D. *Blood Purification*, 41(1–3): 130–4. Epub 15 January 2016.

Yang, Y., Peng, N. et al. (2022). Interaction between smoking and diabetes in relation to subsequent risk of cardiovascular events. *Cardiovascular Diabetology*, 21: 14.

Chapter 8

Barnard, K.D., Young, A.J. & Waugh, N.R. (2010). Self-monitoring of blood glucose: a survey of diabetes UK members with type 2 diabetes who use SMBG. *BMC Research Notes*, 3: 318.

Bener, A. & Yousafzai, M.T. (2014). Effect of Ramadan fasting on diabetes mellitus: a population-based study in Qatar. *Journal* of the *Egyptian Public Health Association*, 89(2): 47–52.

Bryant, K.B., Sheppard, P. et al. (2020). Impact of self-monitoring of blood pressure on processes of hypertension care and long-term blood pressure control. *Journal of the American Heart Association*, 9: e016174.

Carlson, A.L., Daniel, T.D. et al. (2022). Flash glucose monitoring in type 2 diabetes managed with basal insulin in the USA: a retrospective real-world chart review study and meta-analysis. *BMJ Open Diabetes Research & Care*, 10(1): e002590.

Clar, C., Barnard, K. et al. (2010). Self-monitoring of blood glucose in type 2 diabetes: systematic review. *Health Technology Assessment*, 14(12): 1–140.

Diabetes UK (2017). Position statement: self-monitoring of blood glucose (SMBG) for adults with type 2 diabetes. Retrieved from: https://diabetes-resources-production.s3-eu-west-1.amazonaws.com/diabetes-storage/migration/pdf/SMBGType2%2520Final%2520April%25202017.pdf (last reviewed March 2017).

Hui, E., Bravis, V. et al. (2010). Management of people with diabetes wanting to fast during Ramadan. *BMJ*, 340: c3053.

Huygens, M.W.J., Swinkels, I.C.S. et al. (2017). Self-monitoring of health data by patients with a chronic disease: does disease controllability matter? *BMC Family Practice*, 18, article 40.

Li, R., Liang, N. et al. (2020). The effectiveness of self-management of hypertension in adults using mobile health: systematic review and meta-analysis. *JMIR mHealth uHealth*, 8(3): e17776.

Martinez, M., Santamarina, J. et al. (2021). Glycemic variability and cardiovascular disease in patients with type 2 diabetes. *BMJ Open Diabetes Research & Care*, 9: e002032.

McManus, R.J., Mant, J. et al. (2018). Efficacy of self-monitored blood pressure, with or without telemonitoring, for titration of anti-hypertensive medication (TASMINH4): an unmasked randomised controlled trial. *The Lancet*, 391(10124): 948–59.

Orji, R., Lomotey, R. et al. (2018). Tracking feels oppressive and 'punishy': exploring the costs and benefits of self-monitoring for health and wellness. *Digital Health*, 4, January–December.

Schnell, O., Alawi, H. et al. (2013). Self-monitoring of blood glucose in type 2 diabetes: recent studies. *Journal of Diabetes Science and Technology*, 7(2): 478–88.

Tomah, S., Mahmoud, N. et al. (2019). Frequency of self-monitoring of blood glucose in relation to weight loss and A1C during intensive multidisciplinary weight management in patients with type 2 diabetes and obesity. *BMJ Open Diabetes Research & Care*, 7: e000659.

Chapter 9

Alejandro, E.U., Mamerto, T.P. et al. (2020). Gestational diabetes mellitus: a harbinger of the vicious cycle of diabetes. *International Journal of Molecular Sciences*, 21(14): 5003.

Bably, M.B., Paul, R. et al. (2021). Factors associated with the initiation of added sugar among low-income young children participating in the special supplemental nutrition program for women, infants, and children in the US. *Nutrients*, 13(11): 3888.

British Dental Association (2022). British Dental Association market analysis research reveals high levels of sugar in infant foods marketed at babies under 12 months old [press release]. Retrieved from: https://bda.org/news-centre/press-releases/Pages/As-sugary-as-Cola-Dentists-call-for-sweeping-action-on-baby-pouches.aspx.

Che, X., Chen, Z. et al. (2021). Dietary interventions: a promising treatment for polycystic ovary syndrome. *Annals of Nutrition and Metabolism*, 77: 313–23.

Clark, K.A., Alves, J.M. et al. (2020). Dietary fructose intake and hippocampal structure and connectivity during childhood. *Nutrients*, 12(4): 909.

Damm, P., Houshmand-Oeregaard, A. et al. (2016). Gestational diabetes mellitus and long-term consequences for mother and offspring: a view from Denmark. *Diabetologia*, 59: 1396–99.

Desai, M., Jellyman, J.K. & Ross, M.G. (2015). Epigenomics, gestational programming and risk of metabolic syndrome. *International Journal of Obesity*, 39: 633–41.

Deswal, R., Narwal, V. et al. (2020). The prevalence of polycystic ovary syndrome: a brief systematic review. *Journal of Human Reproductive Sciences*, 13(4): 261–71. Epub 28 December 2020.

Goran, M., Plows, J. & Ventura, E. (2019). Effects of consuming sugars and alternative sweeteners during pregnancy on maternal and child health: evidence for a secondhand sugar effect. *Proceedings of the Nutrition Society*, 78(3): 262–71.

Goran, M.I., Martin, A.A. et al. (2017). Fructose in breast milk is positively associated with infant body composition at 6 months of age. *Nutrients*, 9(2): 146.

Herrick, K.A., Fryar, C.D. et al. (2019). Added sugars intake among US infants and toddlers. *Journal of the Academy of Nutrition and Dietetics*, 120(1): 23–32.

Ling, C. & Rönn, T. (2019). Epigenetics in human obesity and type 2 diabetes. *Cell Metabolism*, 29(5): 1028–44.

Plows, J.F., Stanley, J.L. et al. (2018). The pathophysiology of gestational diabetes mellitus. *International Journal of Molecular Sciences*, 19(11): 3342.

UK National Institute for Clinical Health and Excellence (NICE) (2015). Diabetes in pregnancy: management from preconception to the postnatal period, NICE guideline [NG3], 25 February (last updated 16 December 2020). Retrieved from: www.nice.org.uk/guidance/ng3/chapter/Recommendations.

UK NHS Digital (2021). National pregnancy in diabetes audit report 2020. Retrieved from: https://digital.nhs.uk/data-and-information/publications/statistical/national-pregnancy-in-diabetes-audit/2019-and-2020.

Vounzoulaki, E., Khunti, K. et al. (2020). Progression to type 2 diabetes in women with a known history of gestational diabetes: systematic review and meta-analysis. *BMJ*, 369: m1361.

Wang, Y., Wang, K. et al. (2022). Maternal consumption of ultra-processed foods and subsequent risk of offspring overweight or obesity: results from three prospective cohort studies. *BMJ*, 379: e071767.

Weiss, R., Bremer, A.A. & Lustig, R.H. (2013). What is metabolic syndrome, and why are children getting it? *Annals of the New York Academy of Sciences*, 1281: 123–40.

Xie, W., Wang, Y. et al. (2022). Association of gestational diabetes mellitus with overall and type specific cardiovascular and cerebrovascular diseases: systematic review and meta-analysis. *BMJ*, 378: e070244.

Chapter 10

Beck, A.T. (1975). *Cognitive Therapy and the Emotional Disorders*. Madison, CT: International Universities Press, Inc.

Lejuez, C.W., Hopko, D. et al. (2011). Ten year revision of the brief behavioural activation treatment for depression: revised treatment manual. *Behaviour Modification*, 35(2): 111–61.

Myles, P. & Shafran, R. (2016). *The CBT Handbook*. London: Robinson.

Nezu, A.M. & Nezu, C.M. (2019). *Emotion-Centred Problem-Solving Therapy: Treatment Guidelines*. New York: Springer.

Chapter 11

Hudson, J.L. & Moss-Morris, R. (2019). Treating illness distress in chronic illness: integrating mental health approaches with illness self-management. *European Psychologist*, 24(1): 26–37.

Kreider, K.E. (2017). Diabetes distress or major depressive disorder? A practical approach to diagnosing and treating psychological comorbidities of diabetes. *Diabetes Therapy*, 8(1): 1–7.

Pennebaker, J.W. (1997). Writing about emotional experiences as a therapeutic process. *Psychological Science*, 8(3): 162–6.

Watkins, E.R. (2018). *Rumination-Focused Cognitive-Behavioral Therapy for Depression*. New York: The Guilford Press.

Appendix 2: Terminology

Chapter 1

1.1

For more explanation around HbA1c, follow the link to the Diabetes UK website: www.diabetes.co.uk/what-is-hba1c.html

1.2

Commonly used measures to assess 'healthy' body weight

Body mass index (BMI)

BMI is the most widely used measure of weight in relation to health. A standard formula involving height and weight produces a double-digit number which falls into one of several categories. The main categories are low weight, healthy weight, overweight and obese. BMI is a number and a guide only, not a measure of body fat – though it reasonably connects with that, and with the risk of a range of diseases.

The calculation to produce BMI is:

In kg and metres: weight in kg divided by height in m^2. For a person of weight 75.0kg and height 1.83m, this would be $75.0 \div 3.35$ (or 1.83^2) = BMI of 22.4.

In pounds and inches: weight in pounds multiplied by 703 divided by height in inches squared.

For a person of weight 160 pounds and height 65 inches, this would be $160 \times 703 \div 4{,}225\ (65^2) =$ BMI of 26.6.

BMI categories numerically are:

- Below 18.5: under/low weight.

- 18.5–24.9: healthy weight.

- 25.0-29.9: overweight.

- Above 30.0: obese.

The key things to remember about BMI are that: it's a measure of size, not health; it is not a measure of fat – just bulk or mass.

It's possible to be overweight and healthy, and conversely lean and unhealthy. Athletes who carry a lot of lean muscle tissue but little fat can be categorised (wrongly) as overweight and potentially unhealthy.

Also, the connection between BMI and health varies across different ethnicities – people of Asian ethnicity tend to have a higher percentage of body fat and disease risk at the same BMI as a white Caucasian person. The opposite applies with people of Black ethnicity who carry more muscle and less fat at the same BMI.

For more on BMI and related topics, check the two links below from the UK NHS and the US CDC:

www.nhs.uk/live-well/healthy-weight/bmi-calculator/

www.cdc.gov/healthyweight/assessing/bmi/index.html

Waist to height ratio

The other way of assessing body size and risk is to compare your waist and height measurement. Ideally your waist measurement will be less than a half, or 0.5, in whatever units you use. For example, a person who is 5 feet 10 inches, or 70 inches (178cm), tall should have a waist measurement of less than 35 inches (89cm).

Readings above a half or 0.5, especially if over 0.6, correlate with increased abdominal fat and risk of disease. For the example above, 0.6 would be 42 inches waist size.

You can use both BMI and waist to height ratio, though we think that for T2D risk, waist to height is the better measure. The British Heart Foundation magazine, *Heart Matters*, has a good explanation of why waist size matters and how to measure it properly: https://www.bhf.org.uk/informationsupport/heart-matters-magazine/medical/measuring-your-waist

Chapter 2

2.1

Macronutrients (macros) – the basics and some terms unpicked

Macronutrients are so called because they are the large (macro) components of food from which we get our sources of energy and materials for construction and repair of body tissues. The handling of macros in the body is a large part of metabolism.

Proteins are of both plant and animal origin. They are made from amino acids and return to amino acids after digestion. During metabolism, they are mainly channelled into structures for growth and repair, and into the systems that regulate body processes – insulin, for example, is a protein. The largest solid bulk of the human body is protein. Only a small amount of energy that we burn comes from protein, and most authorities recommend a maximum of around 15 per cent of daily calorie intake as protein, which is what many of us eat. A recommended intake of around 0.8g/kg body weight (US/UK) means most of us exceed this.

Protein key points:

- The body can adapt to taking more protein, which can help athletes, people who exercise a lot, and those with extra needs such as debilitating illness, recovery from severe physical trauma and wound healing.

- Protein metabolism itself uses up quite a lot of energy so taking a few more calories as protein can help weight management.

- However, too much will always be converted to glucose, and too much of that will end up as fat. Protein bars and shakes are as likely to end up around your middle as in your muscles! A balance has to be found.

Common protein-rich foods are meat, poultry, fish, milk, yoghurt, cheese, eggs, nuts and seeds. Whilst meat and fish are the richest food sources of protein, you can easily get adequate amounts of protein in your diet if you are vegetarian or vegan.

Several amino acids are essential in food as the body cannot make them. For vegetarian/vegan eaters it's important to have a *variety* of plant protein sources to minimise the risk of missing essential amino acids.

Fats

Dietary fats come from both plant and animal sources and, like carbohydrates, are made from carbon, hydrogen and oxygen. Fat is energy-dense (more than twice the yield of energy per gram compared to protein and carbohydrate) and a primary fuel source for our cells. It contributes, like protein, to the structural and chemical needs of the body. Cholesterol is a type of fat, and a key component of cell structure and nerve tissue (the brain). It's also the building block of many hormones, vital for health and wellbeing.

Triglyceride (TG) is the term for the main type of fat in food, and the main storage fat of the body. Its name comes from the linking up of three fatty acids to a molecule of glycerol. Just as glucose and amino acids are the basic structures of carbohydrates and proteins, fatty acids are the building blocks of fats used as fuel by our cells. Triglycerides are sometimes called triacylglycerols (TAGs). TGs are the same as TAGs.

Foods that are rich sources of fat (TGs) include dairy products (e.g. butter, cheese, cream), meat, oily fish, edible and cooking oils, avocados and nuts. As with proteins, vegetarians and vegans can manage their fat sources to ensure adequacy.

There are essential dietary fatty acids which have to be consumed as the body cannot make them. Fats, like proteins, are therefore essential in the diet. Essential fatty acids are also known as omega fatty acids, a chemical structure term. The terms saturated and unsaturated fats refer to the chemical bonds within the fatty acids they contain.

Fat key points:

- Dietary fat's dual roles are supplying energy, and material for structure and chemical manufacture.

- Saturated fat has been linked with health risks, and though the link seems to be weakening, we are still advised to eat less than 10 per cent of our daily calories as saturated fat.

- Saturated fats tend to be solid at room temperature and are generally of animal origin. Unsaturated fats are mainly oils and of plant origin.

- All foods containing fat have a mixture of saturated and unsaturated fat, so food choices are about the balance of fat that they contain.

- Fat soluble vitamins, such as A, D, E and K can only be absorbed when fat is eaten.

As you can see, terminology and chemistry of fats is complex!

Carbohydrates

Carbohydrates (carbs) are of plant origin and make up the bulk of the foods we are most familiar with. Carbohydrates are nearly all digested down to glucose whether the source be white flour pizza dough, wholegrain pasta or a baked potato – it all ends up as glucose in the body! The exception being the simple sugar fructose, which is covered in Chapter 6.

Glucose is one of the two main fuels for the cells of the body, and the one used for immediate needs. Its storage form, glycogen (mainly in liver and muscle), provides a short-term energy cache for exercise and short fasts.

A *simple* carbohydrate is often also called a sugar. The most common examples are glucose (the universal fuel of life), lactose (found in milk) and fructose (the sugar in fruit). See Chapter 6.

A *complex* carbohydrate is a long chain of simpler sugars, making a bigger structure, for example the energy storage carbohydrate of starch in plants or glycogen in animals. Fibre is mainly formed of indigestible complex carbohydrates.

A 'refined carbohydrate' is one that has undergone significant alteration between the natural form and what's in the food end product. Common examples would be white rice, white flour or bread, where in production the natural grain has been stripped of its outer husk, reducing the nutritional goodness (including fibre) of the grain.

Refined sugar is extracted from sugar cane or beet and turned into sucrose or other similar sweetening products. Man-made sugars lack the natural 'wrappings' – mainly fibre – that make natural products like fruits easier to digest and safer to metabolise.

Refining is really a food manufacturing term and refers to something which is man-made or man-modified for reasons of preservation, presentation or flavouring. It is a substantial part of food processing.

Foods rich in refined carbs and added sugars are what people mean when they say 'bad' or 'unhealthy' carbs. Unrefined, more natural carbs being 'good' or 'healthy' carbs.

Common carb-rich foods are potatoes, pasta, rice, bread, cereals, grains and all sugary things – baked goods, confectionery, sugar-sweetened drinks and many fruits. These are the body's ready sources of fuel to-go – glucose. If you are vegetarian or vegan, carbohydrates offer an easy and wide range of food choices.

A macro summary

Food group	Immediate energy	Storage energy	Building material
Proteins	low	✓	✓✓
Carbohydrates	✓✓	✓	low
Fats	✓	✓✓	✓✓

'Standard nutritional advice' has moulded the intake of our main nutrients over the last forty years. The body will naturally settle on a protein intake making up around 12–20 per cent of daily calories; it might be as low as 5–10 per cent, or as high as 20–25 per cent in some of us, but around 15 per cent is typical. Since around 1980, therefore, guidance on capping dietary fat at around 30 per cent of energy intake has obligated us to take most of our calories (around 55 per cent) as carbohydrate.

Neither carbohydrates nor fats are 'bad' for us – the body is perfectly well equipped to deal with the glucose and fatty acids that they yield. It's possible, however, that increasing our carbohydrate intake is contributing to rising insulin resistance, which is driving up T2D.

Chapter 6

6.1
Glycaemic index and glycaemic load

Glycaemic index (GI)

Glycaemic means 'relating to blood glucose' and glycaemic index, or GI, is a way of rating carbohydrate-containing foods in relation to how much 50g of carbohydrate causes the blood glucose (and insulin) level to rise when that food is eaten on its own.

High GI foods are almost the same as refined, or 'bad', carbs. Lower GI foods are generally regarded as healthier because of their lower insulin response and smaller rise in blood glucose.

Examples of high GI foods are sugar and sugary foods, sugary soft drinks, white bread, potatoes and white rice. Some lower GI examples are wholegrain foods, vegetables, beans and lentils.

Glycaemic load (GL)

GL is a measure that considers the amount of carbohydrate in a portion of food together with how quickly it raises blood glucose levels. In other words it can give a more accurate picture of a food's real-life impact on blood glucose. For example melon, considered a high GI food, has a low GL rating. Fifty grams of carbohydrate in a melon can be almost the whole fruit, whereas a typical portion size is a small fraction of that and, being mainly water, it impacts blood glucose much less than its GI rating might suggest. GI is a more theoretical rating and GL rather more practical.

The abbreviations GI and GL appear often in T2D-related nutritional advice.

There is a good visual explanation of GI and GL here: https://www.youtube.com/watch?v=rOPHv5YKvh4

6.2
Sugar and food labels

The more you read, the more confusing the term sugar becomes! Sugar is the term used in science for simple carbohydrates. The food industry uses the term more or less the same way – so every simple carbohydrate can appear as a sugar on your food label. This commonly causes confusion in dairy-land where unsweetened dairy products – like milk and plain yoghurt – are labelled as containing sugar(s) – though this is lactose which ends up in the body as glucose in adults – just like nearly all carbohydrates!

Most people use the term sugar to mean sucrose (table sugar), which is a chemical combination of glucose and fructose; the reason for being 'sugar-aware' is to limit the consumption of *fructose*. Can we tell how much fructose we might be consuming from reading food labels? Not so easily!

Unsweetened dairy foods are fructose-free, so discount them. 'Free' sugars (UK term) or 'added' sugars (US term) can be assumed to contain fructose as they will be either sucrose or something similar like high fructose corn syrup. These mostly come from processed food and sugar-sweetened beverages; some will be from 'natural' sources like honey or fruit juices – but they will all contain fructose.

Good luck with food labels, which vary a little from place to place. We think if you can get the hang of sugar labelling you've cracked the main part!

Here are some links on sugar labelling that you might find useful. From the US Food and Drug Administration – on 'added sugars' (content from May 2022): https://www.fda.gov/food/new-nutrition-facts-label/added-sugars-new-nutrition-facts-label

From the British Nutrition Foundation (content from June 2021): https://www.nutrition.org.uk/healthy-sustainable-diets/starchy-foods-sugar-and-fibre/sugar/?level=Consumer

Chapter 9

9.1
Epigenetics

A brief summary of the principles from the Virtual Genetics Education Centre, University of Leicester, UK. Most explanations are difficult to follow for non-scientists. This one is a bit easier: https://le.ac.uk/vgec/topics/genetics-and-ethics-and-law/epigenetics

Appendix 3: Resources

Chapter 3

3.1

Link to Jennifer Grayson's podcast, *On the Hadza and Human Metabolism*. An interview with evolutionary biologist Herman Pontzer from 12 March 2019:

www.jennifergrayson.com/uncivilizepodcast/on-the-hadza-and-human-metabolism-herman-pontzer

We hear how scientists had assumed that more active (hunter-gatherer) people, like the Hadza, would burn much more energy living as they do, compared to more typical modern humans with more sedentary lifestyles. The fact they do not was a big surprise, and caused a scientific re-think – for some – on how the body manages its energy. Findings have been confirmed in different populations and in different species. Primates in zoos burn the same calories as those living in the wild.

It may be that homeostatic mechanisms constrain energy expenditure – at least on average over long time periods. This is one of the bigger pieces in the jigsaw of understanding metabolism and energy balance; it confirms that being active is good for us, and should help to make us more healthy – but it probably won't make us leaner.

Chapter 4

Sleep Diary

ACTIVITIES		
A	–	each alcoholic drink
C	–	each caffeinated drink, including coffee, tea, chocolate, cola
P	–	every time you take a sleeping pill
M	–	meals
S	–	snacks
X	–	exercise
T	–	use of toilet during sleep time
N	–	noise that disturbs your sleep
W	–	time of wake-up alarm (if any)
SLEEP TIME (including naps)		
↓	–	mark with a 'down' arrow each time you got into bed
↑	–	mark with an 'up' arrow each time you got out of bed
——	–	mark with a line the time you began and the time you ended your sleep; then join the lines to indicate sleep periods
——	–	mark with a line the time you began and the time you ended any naps, either in the chair or in bed; then join up lines with a broken line to indicate nap periods

Note down any events that influenced your sleep

Example

	p.m.				midnight / a.m.												noon / p.m.					
	6	7	8	9	10	11	12	1	2	3	4	5	6	7	8	9	10	11	12	1	2	3	4	5	6
Activities	A	A	A		S						T				W	S			M		S		M		
Sleep Time							→				←	→				←									

LIGHTS OUT _12.30_ a.m.

TOTAL SLEEP TIME _6_ hrs

Week 1

		p.m.						midnight / a.m.															noon / p.m.				
	6	7	8	9	10	11	12	1	2	3	4	5	6	7	8	9	10	11	12	1	2	3	4	5	6
Activities																										
Sleep Time																										

LIGHTS OUT_____ a.m. / p.m.   TOTAL SLEEP TIME_____ hrs

		p.m.						midnight / a.m.															noon / p.m.				
	6	7	8	9	10	11	12	1	2	3	4	5	6	7	8	9	10	11	12	1	2	3	4	5	6
Activities																										
Sleep Time																										

LIGHTS OUT_____ a.m. / p.m.   TOTAL SLEEP TIME_____ hrs

		p.m.						midnight / a.m.															noon / p.m.				
	6	7	8	9	10	11	12	1	2	3	4	5	6	7	8	9	10	11	12	1	2	3	4	5	6
Activities																										
Sleep Time																										

LIGHTS OUT_____ a.m. / p.m.   TOTAL SLEEP TIME_____ hrs

		p.m.						midnight / a.m.															noon / p.m.				
	6	7	8	9	10	11	12	1	2	3	4	5	6	7	8	9	10	11	12	1	2	3	4	5	6
Activities																										
Sleep Time																										

LIGHTS OUT_____ a.m. / p.m.   TOTAL SLEEP TIME_____ hrs

	6	7	8	9	10	11	12	1	2	3	4	5	6
Activities													
Sleep Time													

LIGHTS OUT _____ a.m. / p.m.   TOTAL SLEEP TIME _____ hrs

	6	7	8	9	10	11	12	1	2	3	4	5	6
Activities													
Sleep Time													

LIGHTS OUT _____ a.m. / p.m.   TOTAL SLEEP TIME _____ hrs

	6	7	8	9	10	11	12	1	2	3	4	5	6
Activities													
Sleep Time													

LIGHTS OUT _____ a.m. / p.m.   TOTAL SLEEP TIME _____ hrs

Reproduced from Anderson, *How to Beat Insomnia and Sleep Problems* (2023), with permission from Little, Brown Book Group.

The National Sleep Foundation, https://www.thensf.org, provides lots of helpful information around the importance of sleep, including how sleep works and how much sleep we need. See Figure 4.1 in Chapter 4.

4.2
Caffeine's connection to sleep problems

Guide to the amount of caffeine in various drinks:

https://www.sleepfoundation.org/caffeine-and-sleep

4.3
Sleep apps

The National Institute for Health and Care Excellence (NICE) has recommended the Sleepio app as an effective alternative to sleeping pills (www.sleepio.com). The app is free for NHS and health and care staff in Scotland. Sleepstation is a clinically validated sleep improvement programme that aims to help people sleep better after just four sessions (www.sleepstation.org.uk). It is possible to apply for free access to the app via the NHS.

Sleepful (www.sleepful.me) is also free to use, appears to be well evidenced and is produced by a reputable academic team. It's well worth a look.

Chapter 5

Below are links to two videos on achieving remission of T2D against the odds.

5.1
Eric and Peety

Possibly the most engaging and moving short film on T2D you could expect to see. It's the story of Eric, who had T2D and was metabolically unwell and grossly overweight, and his dog Peety, also middle-aged and overweight. Eric's doctor had told him to invest in a funeral plaque as he was soon going to need one. A nutritionist suggested getting a rescue dog – and we see how Eric and Peety came together to rescue each other. It's guaranteed to have you reaching for the tissues, then maybe your walking or running shoes! A book is available too – *Walking with Peety*.

https://www.youtube.com/watch?v=Rm0qYRWQpZI

5.2

Fixing Dad

A BBC documentary about how one family tackled T2D. A story about putting T2D into remission, about finding the motivation and grit to make something work, and the family love underpinning it. It is inspiring. There is also a book of the same name – both film and book were a family effort.

https://www.youtube.com/watch?v=ghSkYZu0tvI

Fixing Dad and *Eric and Peety* show us that the wellspring of motivation is more important than any other single thing when facing a big challenge to health.

5.3

Taylor, R. (2020). *Life Without Diabetes: The Definitive Guide to Understanding and Reversing Your Type 2 Diabetes*. London: Short Books.

An accessible explanation of how T2D comes about from one of the people who actually worked it out. Chapter 7 of the book focuses on reversal using a very low-calorie diet.

5.4
Some guidance on 800kcal per day eating for T2D reversal

1. Professor Roy Taylor's book (see above) gives guidance on the practical aspects of reversing T2D, as well as a lengthy section on foods to help with the initial 800kcal/day of the very low-calorie approach. There are also recipe ideas to help with the gradual increasing of calories for the longer term. A major plus is that many of the recipes have been devised by people participating in the research study which pioneered this dietary approach.

2. Look online for 200kcal-per-meal replacement foods/ shakes. There are many. This is just one we checked more or less at random (no affiliations). They are UK-based but have outlets in some European countries and the US: https://www. theproteinworks.com. The replacement food products are very varied and, based on around 200kcal per serving (four per day), they seem economical. Full micronutrient profiles are shown for selected products. All seem to be matched to give at least the daily recommended levels, so no need for extra supplements. They give a good daily protein and fibre intake for the 800kcal daily target. There are several vegan options which are equally balanced nutritionally for a very low-calorie phase in T2D reversal.

3. For milk options, the best is skimmed cow's milk, so not helpful for vegans. For 800kcal per day, 2.3 litres of milk (four pints, or eight cups) gives adequate protein at 80g per day. Other milk options, such as full-fat dairy or oat milk, would be too low in protein. Semi-skimmed dairy and unsweetened soy might be a little low without supplementation – personal nutritional advice would be needed. A multivitamin and some roughage are recommended.

There are also multiple 200kcal-per-meal recipe books and recipe options accessible online. As far as fluids go, drinking water steadily throughout the day to stay hydrated and manage thirst is all that's needed. Tea and coffee are OK (allowing for milk calories, if added). Herbal/flavoured teas are good.

Alcohol is best minimised or avoided in the early phase of this approach, which might help reset your relationship with alcohol long-term. For all very low-calorie options, we would strongly recommend checking the details with your T2D dietician or nutritionist.

5.5

This is a presentational version by the late Dr Sarah Hallberg of the paper cited in Appendix 1 under Chapter 5 – much more engaging to see and hear her views on T2D reversal and diet. A powerful challenge to standard nutritional advice:

https://www.youtube.com/watch?v=da1vvigy5tQ

Chapter 6

6.1
Food diary
See table opposite.

6.2
A beginner's guide to mindful eating from Healthline:
https://www.healthline.com/nutrition/mindful-eating-guide

6.3
Another Healthline contribution – this time on the Mediterranean Diet. There are a number of other helpful links, too.

Mediterranean Diet 101: A Meal Plan and Beginner's Guide
https://www.healthline.com/nutrition/mediterranean-diet-meal-plan

6.4
Connecting sugar with metabolic syndrome and processed food. Two video presentations by Dr Robert Lustig, widely and highly regarded as a leading expert on child health and metabolism, and a fierce critic of sugar and processed food. Both are highly relevant to T2D. Don't worry about following it all – most folk have to watch more than once to pick things up!

https://www.youtube.com/watch?v=zx-QrilOoSM – for metabolic syndrome.

and

https://www.youtube.com/watch?v=pvgxNDuQ5DI&t=2525s – for processed food.

Food diary

	Monday	Tuesday	Wednesday	Thursday	Friday	Saturday	Sunday
Breakfast							
Morning							
Lunch							
Afternoon							
Tea/Dinner							
Evening							

6.5

The low-carbohydrate world in current medical practice

A low-carbohydrate information pack and access to multiple resources, including food guidance, are in the following links, both highly recommended:

Information for people with T2D, used in the UK General Practice of Dr David Unwin:

https://phcuk.org/wp-content/uploads/A_5_page_low_carb_diet_leaflet_Unwin_2021-converted.pdf

And an interesting and informative resource on low-carbohydrate food choices produced by the New Forest Primary Care Network UK:

https://newforestpcn.co.uk/low-carb/

Chapter 7

7.1

A medication guide for common drugs used in T2D

Note: this is not a treatment guide, simply an outline of what's available. The treatment route is through shared decision-making between yourself and your healthcare team.

Medicine Type	Option	Form	Impact on Weight	Risk of Hypoglycaemia
Metformin	Metformin	Tablet	None	Low
Pioglitazone	Pioglitazone	Tablet	Gain	Low
DPP-4 Inhibitor ('Gliptins')	Alogliptin, Linagliptin, Sitagliptin, Saxagliptin, Vildagliptin	Tablet	None	Low
Sulphonylureas ('SUs')	Gliclazide, Glimepiride, Glipizide, Tolbutamide	Tablet	Gain	Moderate (High in older people)
SGLT2 Inhibitor ('Flozins')	Canagliflozin, Dapagliflozin, Empagliflozin, Ertugliflozin	Tablet	Loss	Low

Note: First-line choices are usually from this group. Some first-line medicines can be second-line choices depending on the overall route plan.

These are usually second-line options

Medicine Type	Option	Form	Impact on Weight	Risk of Hypoglycaemia
GLP-1	Dulaglutide, Exenatide, Liraglutide, Lixisenatide, Semaglutide	Tablet or injection	Loss	Low
Insulin	Insulin options	Injection	Gain	High

Note: All drugs carry cautions for dose adjustment (or avoidance) in kidney or liver impairment. Pioglitazone should be avoided in liver impairment. The GLP-1 group have specific cautions for use in people with severe bowel or stomach conditions.

7.2

An example 'decision aid' for increasing treatment in T2D and working with HbA1c targets in T2D:

https://www.nice.org.uk/guidance/ng28/update/ng28-update-3/documents/supporting-documentation-3

7.3

Patient education: Quitting smoking (Beyond the Basics). A US-based summary of the medical help available for stopping smoking – but widely applicable and up to date.

https://www.uptodate.com/contents/quitting-smoking-beyond-the-basics

7.4

More on smoking cessation. A simple explanation, with tips on stopping smoking by Professor Robert West of UCL, and supportive of using temporary nicotine replacement:

https://www.youtube.com/watch?v=0lBqv41OneM

7.5

Practising nasal breathing (in) – a simple and relaxing way to increase nitric oxide production. There are numerous demonstrations on YouTube. This one is easy to follow:

https://www.youtube.com/watch?v=8vN08IuParo

7.6

For anyone interested in learning more about glucosamine, this recent review article could be a start. Note that glucosamine has to be taken for many weeks to achieve any noticeable benefit, and months/long-term to maintain that. We would suggest a symptom diary to help judge this.

To provide benefit, glucosamine doses may need to be around 1500mg per day or more.

Glucosamine is often taken with chondroitin sulphate and many preparations contain both.

Chondroitin may also reduce inflammation and promote cartilage health. The dose range in the various preparations is wide, and it's hard to advise on this. Chondroitin has the potential for side-effects (gastrointestinal), though these are reported to be mild; ask for advice from a pharmacist or doctor, especially if you are on an anticoagulant (in which case, maybe best avoided).

Conrozier, T. & Lohse, T. (2022). Glucosamine as a treatment for osteoarthritis: what if it's true? *Frontiers in Pharmacology*, 13, 17 March: 820971.

Chapter 8

8.1
Blank page-a-day self-monitoring diary, for copying/use, on page 436.

8.2

A visual demonstration of self-monitoring of blood glucose –
we liked this one best:

https://www.youtube.com/watch?v=eOsY84oYqKg

Alternatively, use this from Diabetes UK:

https://www.youtube.com/watch?v=H5uXed6TBlM

Or, of course, speak to your healthcare team.

8.3

'Sick day rules' for T2D – simple to follow. Written with
COVID-19 in mind but applicable to self-management of any
common illness at home:

https://www.england.nhs.uk/london/wp-content/uploads/
sites/8/2020/04/3.-Covid-19-Type-2-Sick-Day-Rules-Crib-
Sheet-06042020.pdf

8.4

Ramadan and T2D advice will be available by country from
your healthcare team. Here, for example, are factsheets from
Diabetes UK:

https://diabetes-resources-production.s3.eu-west-1.amazon
aws.com/resources-s3/public/2023-02/Ramadan%20factsheet
%202023.pdf

And the Muslim Council of Britain:

https://mcb.org.uk/wp-content/uploads/2022/11/Ramadan-
Factsheet-English-2015-9_3_15.pdf

Blank page-a-day self-monitoring diary, for copying/use

Page a Day: Self-Monitoring Diary for T2D

Date:

Breakfast	Blood Glucose	Activity/Exercise:
	Before:	
	Time:	
	After:	
	Time:	

Lunch	Blood Glucose	Sleep:
	Before:	Number of Hours:
	Time:	Sleep Quality: (1 = Poor, 5 = Excellent)
	After:	1 2 3 4 5
	Time:	

Tea/Dinner	Blood Glucose	Mood/Tension:
	Before: Time: After: Time:	Mood: (1 = Very low, 5 = Good/Happy) 1 2 3 4 5 Tension: (1 = Calm/Relaxed, 5 = Very Stressed) 1 2 3 4 5

Drinks and Snacks	Symptoms, Issues and Problems

Reminders for the Day	Measurements
	Blood pressure: Time: Weight:

Chapter 9

9.1

Is low-carb safe during pregnancy? YouTube presentation by diabetes educator and dietician Lily Nichols:

https://www.youtube.com/watch?v=u6_CcBQDHMo

There are a number of related presentations/podcasts to peruse too. Lily is renowned for an evidence-based, thorough and sensible approach, and has written books on eating in pregnancy, and for GDM.

9.2

Below is an example comparing a traditional and 'real food' meal plan. A Mediterranean diet with a carbohydrate intake of less than 150g per day is the same sort of thing.

Example	Conventional	Real Food
Breakfast	Oatmeal Strawberries Low-fat milk	Eggs cooked in butter Sautéed kale & mushrooms Tangerine
Lunch/Dinner	Turkey sandwich w/ light mayo Salad Banana Low-fat milk	Grass-fed beef meatballs Spaghetti squash Tomato-cream sauce Broccoli Parmesan cheese

Snack	Carrot slices Wholewheat crackers	Full-fat Greek yoghurt Berries
Dessert	Low-fat frozen yoghurt	Dark chocolate Cashews

Table courtesy of Lily Nichols, RDN, CDE

Chapter 10

10.1

Support agencies

NHS 111 provides urgent care, advice and mental health support 24 hours a day.

Phone: 111

Website: www.111.nhs.uk

Samaritans is a voluntary organisation providing support to people in distress 24 hours a day.

Phone: 116 123

Email: jo@samaritans.org

Website: www.samaritans.org

Childline is a free helpline for anyone under 19 to talk about any issues that they are facing 24 hours a day.

Phone: 0800 111

Website: www.childline.org.uk

Live chat: www.childline.org.uk/get-support/1-2-1-counsellor-chat/

PAPYRUS is a charity for the prevention of young suicide. It offers support and advice 24 hours a day to anyone under 35 at risk of suicide.

Phone: 0800 068 4141

Email: pat@papyrus-uk.org

Website: www.papyrus-uk.org

Shout is a free confidential text messaging service offering support 24 hours a day to anyone who is struggling to cope.

Text: Shout to 85258

Website: www.giveusashout.org

The Mix offers information and support for under 25s 4 p.m.–11 p.m. on its phone line Monday to Friday. They also offer a crisis text service through their website.

Text: THEMIX to 85258

Website: https://www.themix.org.uk

Young Minds provides mental health support to young people in mental health crisis 24 hours a day.

Website: www.youngminds.org.uk

Age UK is a charity providing support for older people every day, 8 a.m.–7 p.m.

Phone: 0800 678 1602

Website: www.ageuk.org.uk

They also provide **Silver Line Helpline**, which operates a 24-hour helpline every day providing support for older people.

Phone: 0800 4 70 80 90

Website: www.thesilverline.org.uk

Breathing Space (Scotland) provides a free support service for anyone in Scotland over 16 who is experiencing low mood, depression or anxiety. As well as a phone service, it offers live web chat from Monday to Friday 6 p.m.–2 a.m. and Saturday and Sunday 4 p.m.–12 a.m.

Phone: 0800 83 85 87 (24 hours at weekends, from Friday 6 p.m.–Monday 6 a.m., and 6 p.m.–2 a.m. weekdays)

Website: www.breathingspace.scot

CALM (Campaign Against Living Miserably) is a charity that offers a helpline and live chat for anyone over 15 every day 5 p.m.–12 a.m.

Phone: 0800 58 58 58

Website: www.thecalmzone.net

Lifeline (Northern Ireland) is a crisis helpline service, operating 24 hours every day, for people in Northern Ireland who are experiencing distress.

Phone: 0808 808 8000

Website: www.lifelinehelpline.info

Mind is a charity that provides advice and support to people experiencing mental health difficulties, Monday to Friday 9 a.m.–5 p.m.

Phone: 0208 215 2243

Email: info@mind.org.uk

Website: www.mind.org.uk

SANELine is a national out-of-hours charity mental health helpline offering emotional support, available every day 4 p.m.–10 p.m.

Phone: 0300 304 7000

Website: www.sane.org.uk

My symptoms of depression

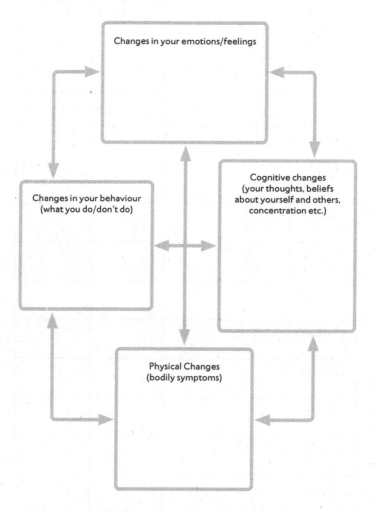

Daily Monitoring Diary

Daily monitoring diary			
Time of Day	Activity	Enjoyment/ Pleasure Rating 0–10	Importance/ Achievement Rating 0–10
6–7 a.m.			
7–8 a.m.			
8–9 a.m.			
9–10 a.m.			
10–11 a.m.			
11–12 p.m.			
12–1 p.m.			
1–2 p.m.			
2–3 p.m.			
3–4 p.m.			
4–5 p.m.			

5–6 p.m.			
6–7 p.m.			
7–8 p.m.			
8–9 p.m.			
9–10 p.m.			
10–11 p.m.			
11–12 a.m.			
12–1 a.m.			
1–2 a.m.			
2–3 a.m.			
3–4 a.m.			
4–5 a.m.			
5–6 a.m.			
Overall mood for the day:			

My Values

Life areas, values and activities

Relationships	
Education/Career/Work	
Recreation/Interests	
Mind/Body/Spirituality	
Regular Responsibilities	

Activity Selection and Ranking

Activity List

Activity	Indicate level of difficulty (1–15)

Activity Schedule

Activity schedule

Instructions: Please write in each box for every hour of the day:
Activity, Achievement (A = 0–10) and Pleasure (P = 0–10)

Time	Monday	Tuesday	Wednesday	Thursday	Friday	Saturday	Sunday
6–7 a.m.							
7–8 a.m.							
8–9 a.m.							
9–10 a.m.							
10–11 a.m.							
11–12 p.m.							
12–1 p.m.							
1–2 p.m.							
2–3 p.m.							

3–4 p.m.								
4–5 p.m.								
5–6 p.m.								
6–7 p.m.								
7–8 p.m.								
8–9 p.m.								
9–10 p.m.								
10–11 p.m.								
11–12 a.m.								
12–1 a.m.								
1–2 a.m.								
2–3 a.m.								
3–4 a.m.								
4–5 a.m.								
5–6 a.m.								

Problem Solving

Step 1. Identify your problem precisely
Step 2. Write down as many possible solutions as you can
Step 3. Think through the pros and cons of each solution

Solution 1.	
Pros	**Cons**

Solution 2.	
Pros	Cons

Solution 3.	
Pros	Cons

Solution 4.	
Pros	Cons

Solution 5.	
Pros	Cons

452 • Living Well With Type 2 Diabetes

Solution 6.	
Pros	Cons

Solution 7.	
Pros	Cons

Solution 8.	
Pros	Cons

Solution 9.	
Pros	Cons

Solution 10.	
Pros	Cons

Step 4. Select the best possible solution

Step 5. Plan how to carry out the solution

Step 6. Put the plan into action

Step 7. Review what happens

Chapter 11

Cost–benefit analysis

Benefits (pros)		Costs (cons)	
Describe	Importance (0–100%)	Describe	Importance (0–100%)

Thinking errors

Thinking error	Description	Example
'All or nothing' or 'black and white' thinking	You do not do things by halves – there is no middle ground or shades of grey. People are either successful or a failure; they either like you or hate you; you are either right or wrong.	
Overgeneralising	You take one specific event and apply it to lots of others in your life; this includes a negative evaluation of yourself.	
Minimising and maximising	You blow things out of proportion, making mountains out of molehills; you underplay and undervalue your strengths but emphasise your weaknesses.	

Fortune-telling	You predict that things will turn out badly, no matter what you say or do.	
Emotional reasoning	You base your judgement of the situation on how you are feeling. You *feel* anxious so you *think* there must be danger.	
Selective abstracting	You focus on one negative aspect of an event rather than taking all aspects into account.	

Discounting the positive	You discount positive things about yourself.	
Personalising	When something goes wrong, you blame yourself. The same is not true when things go right.	
Mind-reading	You think you know what others are thinking. This is very common and usually involves believing they are thinking something bad about you.	

Thought Diary (4-column)

Date	Situation	Emotion	Thought
Include day of week and time of day where relevant	Where were you? What were you doing? Who were you with?	**Rate intensity 0–100%**	What was going through your head just as you started to feel the emotion? List all thoughts and images. **Rate belief 0–100% and circle the most upsetting thought**

Thought Diary (9-column)

Date Include day of week and time of day where relevant	Situation	Emotion **Rate intensity 0–100%**	Thought What was going through your head just as you started to feel the emotion? List all thoughts and images. **Rate belief 0–100% and circle the most upsetting thought**	Evidence for the most upsetting thought	Evidence against the most upsetting thought	Alternative thought and rate belief in it	Re-rate belief in upsetting thought and intensity of emotion	What to do next

Appendix 4: Further reading

Chapter 3

3.1

Lieberman, D.E. (2021). *Exercised: Why Something We Never Evolved to Do Is Healthy and Rewarding.* (US title: *Exercised: The Science of Physical Activity, Rest and Health.*) New York: Pantheon Books.

Professor Daniel Lieberman, a paleoanthropologist at Harvard University, is an expert on the evolution of the human body. His contribution here to understanding the place of exercise in modern human life and health is informative and engaging.

3.2

Further reading on exercise: a quick summary of the benefits from Diabetes UK: https://www.diabetes.org.uk/guide-to-diabetes/managing-your-diabetes/exercise

3.3

UK Chief Medical Officers' Physical Activity Guidelines. If you want something substantive, this is thorough, informative and engaging – for a policy document!

https://assets.publishing.service.gov.uk/government/uploads/
system/uploads/attachment_data/file/832868/uk-chief-medi
cal-officers-physical-activity-guidelines.pdf

Chapter 4

4.1
Anderson, K. (2023). *How to Beat Insomnia and Sleep Problems*.
London: Robinson.

This self-help book offers an easy-to-follow step-by-step guide
to overcoming insomnia using CBT techniques. Dr Anderson
is a consultant neurologist who runs a neurology sleep service
in north-east England and has a clinical and research interest
in all sleep disorders. She also has an excellent TED talk on
sleep: https://www.youtube.com/watch?v=Mr_N-lbg4Rw

4.2
Walker, M. (2018). *Why We Sleep: The New Science of Sleep and
Dreams*. Harlow, UK: Penguin Books.

This is a popular science book about sleep written by Matthew
Walker, an English scientist and director of the Centre for
Human Sleep Science at the University of California, Berkeley.
Professor Walker specialises in neuroscience and psychology
and is regarded as a leading expert on sleep. The book is not
a self-help book but ideal for those wanting to understand
sleep's place as one of the pillars of good health. Also listen to
his podcasts and TED talks.

Chapter 6

6.1

On the machinations of commerce and politics in nutrition and health:

Susan Greenhalgh, research professor at Harvard University, uncovers how, 'through a complex web of institutional, financial, and personal links, Coca-Cola has been able to influence China's health policies'.

Greenhalgh, S. (2019). Making China safe for Coke: how Coca-Cola shaped obesity science and policy in China. Feature article. *BMJ*, 364: k5050.

The online version of the article at www.bmj.com/content/364/bmj.k5050 contains an audio link.

6.2

Writings on the fat/sugar debate which some might find interesting or helpful:

Taubes, G. (2001). The Soft Science of Dietary Fat. *Science*, 291, 30 March.

Meach, R. (2018). From John Yudkin to Jamie Oliver: A Short but Sweet History on the War against Sugar. In: Gentilcore, D. & Smith, M. (eds), *Proteins, Pathologies and Politics: Dietary Innovation and Disease from the Nineteenth Century*. London (UK); New York (NY): Bloomsbury Academic, Chapter 7. Available at: https://www.ncbi.nlm.nih.gov/books/NBK542158/

6.3

Here's some further recommended reading for anyone considering long-term low-carbohydrate eating. Everything you need to know about low-carbohydrate eating from two experienced practitioner-researchers.

Volek, J.S. and Phinney, S.D. (2011). *The Art and Science of Low Carbohydrate Living*. Beyond Obesity LLC.

6.4

Dr Michael Mosley has popularised intermittent fasting, principally through his well-known 5:2 diet and book, with two fasting or low-calorie days per week. More recently he has written about both very low-calorie and very low-carbohydrate approaches. There are several books to peruse. Suggested:

Mosley, M. and Spencer, M. (2014). *The Fast Diet*. London: Short Books Limited. This is an updated version of the original 5:2 book.

Mosley, M. (2021). *The Fast 800 Keto*. London: Short Books Limited. Using a very low-carbohydrate (and very low-calorie) diet to initiate weight loss/reverse T2D, with gradual introduction of carbohydrate, and a low(ish)-carbohydrate Mediterranean diet approach for the long term. Probably the route we would choose ourselves for T2D.

Chapter 7

7.1

Papworth, M. (2023). *How to Beat Fears and Phobias: A Brief, Evidence-based Self-help Treatment.* London: Robinson.

This self-help book offers an easy-to-follow step-by-step guide to overcoming fears and phobias using CBT techniques. Dr Papworth is a clinical psychologist who edits a series of books focusing on how to beat common psychological problems.

7.2

Worrall, J. (2021). *Statins and CVD (Cardio-Vascular Disease): Now It's Personal!* London: LSE.

A thoughtful way of looking at statin use from an individual perspective by John Worrall, emeritus professor, London School of Economics.

https://www.lse.ac.uk/philosophy/blog/2021/06/29/statins-and-cvd-now-its-personal/

7.3

Carr, A. (2015). *Allen Carr's Easy Way to Stop Smoking.* London: Penguin.

First published in 1985, Carr's book remains a self-help classic. It won't help everyone, but it gives another option to the medical route and does not advocate for nicotine replacement therapy. There are numerous updates and variations on the original book.

7.4
Marks, D. (2017). *Stop Smoking Now: A self-help guide using cognitive behavioural techniques* (second edition). London: Robinson.

This week-long programme using techniques from cognitive behavioural therapy (CBT) by David Marks is highly recommended.

Chapter 8

8.1
Suggested reading – especially for those with T2D on insulin:

Brown, A. (2017). *Bright Spots and Landmines*. San Francisco: diaTribe Foundation.

Possibly the best book on T1D from a practical perspective, but much of this book is also applicable to people with T2D – indeed even to people without diabetes. There are four main sections – food, mindset, exercise and sleep – full of reflective thoughts and practical tips. It would be impossible to read this book and not pick up something worth considerably more than its price.

Chapter 9

9.1
Lustig, R. (2021). *Metabolical*. London: Hodder & Stoughton.

Dr Robert Lustig is to the 'internal environment' of bodily health what David Attenborough is to the 'external environment' of planetary health. *Metabolical* is about understanding the mechanisms of chronic disease and the links, in particular with processed food. We may intuitively feel that the modern western diet is both unhealthy and addictive, and Dr Lustig helps us to understand why. As an expert on childhood obesity he is able to pull together for us the links between the food environment and metabolic disease from childhood onwards.

Chapter 10

10.1
Nezu, A., Nezu, C.M. and D'Zurilla, T.J. (2006). *Solving Life's Problems: A 5-Step Guide to Enhanced Wellbeing.* New York: Springer Publishing Company.

The authors of this book are renowned experts in problem-solving therapy. In this book they use a five-step approach.

10.2
Papworth, M. (2023). *How to Beat Depression and Persistent Low Mood: A Brief, Evidence-based Self-help Treatment.* London: Robinson.

This self-help book offers an easy-to-follow step-by-step guide to overcoming depression using behavioural activation. It's written in a friendly and engaging style using case studies to illustrate the use of the approach.

Chapter 11

11.1

Myles, P. and Shafran, R. (2016). *The CBT Handbook: A Comprehensive Guide to Using CBT to Overcome Depression, Anxiety, Stress, Low Self-esteem and Anger*. London: Robinson.

This book has some useful sections on relaxation, cost–benefit analysis, and working with thoughts, with lots of practical exercises throughout as well as diaries and questionnaires to measure progress.

11.2

Pennebaker, J.W. and Smyth, J.M. (2016). *Opening Up by Writing It Down: How Expressive Writing Improves Health and Eases Emotional Pain* (third edition). New York: The Guilford Press.

This book offers a simple yet powerful self-help strategy that is grounded in scientific research. It is written by leading experts who describe how taking a few minutes to write about deeply felt personal experiences or problems can be helpful, including by providing a number of health benefits. There are lots of stories and examples throughout and it includes practical exercises to help you try out expressive writing for yourself.

Index

Page numbers in *italic* refer to Figures and Tables